"I am delighted that there is now ... s-
carriage: The Good News; it is long overdue! I recommend this book to
any of my patients unfortunate enough to have had a miscarriage. It is
informative, well-written, and should be read by any couple contemplating getting pregnant."

—MICHAEL L. BRODMAN, M.D., chairman, Department of
Obstetrics, Gynecology & Reproductive Sciences,
Mount Sinai School of Medicine, New York

"A wonderfully written text which will provide clear, up-to-date explanations for complex medical problems involving recurrent pregnancy
loss. The personal accounts allow us all to be inspired by the desire to
reproduce!"

—ANDREI REBARBER, M.D., clinical associate professor,
Mount Sinai School of Medicine, New York; president,
Maternal Fetal Medicine Associates, PLLC

"Shatters the myth that all miscarriages are unavoidable. A 'take control' self-help book."

—SAMI DAVID, M.D., reproductive endocrinologist, assistant
clinical professor, Mount Sinai School of Medicine, New York

"Dr. Jonathan Scher is so much more than a doctor; he is that rare thing in the medical world: a humanist. *Preventing Miscarriage* should be required reading not only for every woman who has experienced the emotional roller coaster of miscarriage, but also for every ob/gyn who treats them. If more doctors read this book, there would be greater understanding of how to treat women who experience such heartbreaking loss: not just physically, but emotionally. Dr. Scher's wisdom and experience are only matched by his compassion and his desire to help his patients by giving them the most information and the most options. For countless women who previously heard 'there is nothing you can do,' Dr. Scher's book is a beacon of hope. If you are not one of the lucky ones who get to see him for a consultation, then you can do the next best thing: read his book. The mixture of case histories, new scientific evidence, and common sense make it unique among the shelves of fertility books. *Preventing Miscarriage* is an important, groundbreaking book."

—JANINE DI GIOVANNI, contributing editor, *Vanity Fair*;
author of *Madness Visible: A Memoir of War*

"Dr. Scher is extraordinary; his belief in my ability to have twins at 57 was a huge factor in their successful birth. He was not only caring and supportive, but he was also my rock. His medical expertise was exceptional, leaving no stone unturned; his meticulous attention to every detail assured the safe delivery of my miracle twins."

—ALETA ST. JAMES

Preventing Miscarriage

·THE GOOD NEWS·

JONATHAN SCHER, M.D.,

and

CAROL DIX

 Collins

An Imprint of HarperCollins*Publishers*

PREVENTING MISCARRIAGE, REVISED EDITION. Copyright © 2005 by
Jonathan Scher, M.D., and Carol Dix. All rights reserved. Printed in
the United States of America. No part of this book may be used or
reproduced in any manner whatsoever without written permission except
in the case of brief quotations embodied in critical articles and reviews.
For information address HarperCollins Publishers, 10 East 53rd
Street, New York, NY 10022.

HarperCollins books may be purchased for educational, business,
or sales promotional use. For information, please write: Special Markets
Department, HarperCollins Publishers, 10 East 53rd Street,
New York, NY 10022.

First Collins Edition published 2005

Designed by Ellen Cipriano

Library of Congress Cataloging-in-Publication Data is available
upon request.

ISBN-10: 0-06-073481-7

ISBN-13: 978-0-06-073481-7

07 08 09 WBC/RRD 10 9 8 7 6 5 4 3

This book is dedicated to all my patients who had the courage not to take NO for an answer and who never gave up hope in their quest to have children.

CONTENTS

❦

LIST OF ILLUSTRATIONS

ACKNOWLEDGMENTS

I would like to thank my colleagues of the American Society of Reproductive Immunology who by doing their research are expanding our knowledge of the miracle of pregnancy and thereby helping women have children when they might not have done.

Thank you too to my many esteemed colleagues who have referred patients to me and whose enthusiasm has been so valuable to me in this emerging field.

I would like to thank organizations such as the American Fertility Society and Resolve who give support to patients who repeatedly lose their pregnancies through an emotionally devastating experience.

I would also like to thank Carmen Dabao, my professional assistant and right hand for believing in what I do and helping in the care of my patients. Thanks to the rest of my office team, RNs Kathleen Burke and Patricia Prinz, whose help is invaluable.

Special thanks to Laurie Chameides, obstetrical social worker at Mount Sinai Hospital, for helping with references and websites relating to pregnancy loss. Thanks to Paula Koz and Vincent Dabao for the illustrations.

Thanks to Carol Dix, my coauthor, without whom this book

could not have been done. Of course, the gracious help, advice, and patience of our editor at HarperCollins, Toni Sciarra, was so special.

I need to acknowledge the many women and men who have shared their stories with me over the years, including those I interviewed for the first edition of this book and the new edition.

I would like to recognize my partners, Drs. Thomas Kerenyi, Victor Grazi, Andrew Kramer, and Jonathan Lanzkowsky for their professionalism and their support in the care of our patients.

Last but not least, my loyal family, who stand by me in my professional life and during the many hours of commitment to this book. Thank you, my wife, Brenda, daughters, Amanda and Robyn, son-in-law, Nathaniel, and adorable grandchildren, Dylan, Trevor, and Nicole.

᭗

Introduction

Fifteen years have passed since *Preventing Miscarriage: The Good News* was first published in 1990. This is a long time in the development of modern medicine, so medical writer Carol Dix and I have undertaken a total revision of the original work. This newly updated edition of *Preventing Miscarriage* is designed to help women, their husbands and partners, and in some cases their doctors, understand the current treatments available and the level of care and support women should expect if they have experienced miscarriage, pregnancy loss, unexplained infertility, or repeated failure with in vitro fertilization (IVF). We have included the latest medical facts and opinion, as well as recent stories of success.

Since 1990, *Preventing Miscarriage* has gained a following among its readers. Many have written to tell us about their experiences:

֍

"Not only does this book have stories from real women who have gone through the heartbreak and trauma of miscarriage, it also has very practical advice on what you can do to prevent it. It presents technical information in a clearly understood, yet very compassionate manner. I liked this book so much that I recently bought a second copy for a friend."

"*Preventing Miscarriage: The Good News* is the best book I read. It was very informative and supportive too. . . . The information is straightforward. It was easy to understand, and it is a book that can always be used for reference in the future."

"I have read several other books on the subject and have found this one to be most helpful. It is written with a caring voice and includes the most up-to-date information available on the subject."

"When I had my appointment with Dr. Scher, I bought the first edition of this book. I always remember the line that 'miscarriage is something you never forget.' The book made me feel so much better, like I wasn't alone. It became my bible. When he said to me, 'You will have your own baby,' sounding so confident, that just changed everything. That time was so hard. It's really important to have a doctor you can relate to."

֍

Many more couples are having successful pregnancies these days because of the emerging new research and treatment methods available. Women and men need to know what these treatments are; what questions to ask their doctors; and how to ensure that they are being offered the most appropriate treatment, rather than being told to keep on trying again and again.

Pregnancy is an immunological paradox: it is the only circumstance in mammalian nature in which a foreign substance is allowed to grow in the body for an extended period of time. Just think what happens to germs, skin grafts, and organ transplants. Unless our immune system is suppressed, our bodies reject those foreign invaders. Pregnancy is therefore a remarkable and awe-inspiring event.

If the mother's body rejects the fertilized egg, the pregnancy fails. In fact, "unexplained infertility" may be repeated pregnancy loss due to implantation failure. This is an increasingly important area of research. Today a whole new range of maternal immunological tests is available.

Repeat failure of IVF treatments in particular may have an immunologic cause. Patients who repeatedly fail IVF should have certain tests for immune disorders. For example, one cause of implantation failure or rejection may be the mother's own natural killer (NK) cells, which, at an elevated level, may prevent the embryo from implanting in the womb. New immunologic tests now make it possible to measure the mother's NK cells. Radical new emerging treatments to prevent miscarriage include the infusion of intravenous immune globulin (IVIG). Such treatments are at the cutting edge of medicine and are still seen as experimental.

Blood-clotting disorders called *thrombophilias* are another cause of recurrent pregnancy loss (RPL). Six or seven different types of thrombophilia have now been identified. Only a decade ago injected heparin was being used experimentally to treat these thrombophilias. This form of treatment is now widespread, and new generations of heparin are being developed that have a lesser bone thinning effect. (If you are prescribed heparin, you should also take 1500 milligrams of calcium daily and have monthly blood tests.)

Another new area of research and treatment is *histopathology*. Following miscarriage, placental tissue is sent to a placental pathologist to determine the immediate cause of the loss of pregnancy. This tissue is all-important, as it is the connection between mother and fetus. Hospitals in the United States keep the tissue specimens for 20 years. A skilled placental pathologist will be able to review a patient's previous pregnancy losses and form a considered opinion on the source of the problem: whether the miscarriage is due to infection, genetic, immunologic, or blood-flow problems.

Treatment and care of a woman with a history of repeat miscarriages or failed IVF is paramount. When women who have previously miscarried become pregnant again, their pregnancy should be handled as high-risk. They may be at risk for late-pregnancy complications such as growth retardation, preeclampsia, and premature labor. They will certainly be in need of extra support and reassurance from their doctor.

There are many excellent websites and online support groups for women who are undergoing repeat pregnancy loss. These can help women build their knowledge and seek comfort from other women. For a list of websites, see the Resources section at the end of this book.

My interest and involvement in the field of recurrent miscarriage began about twenty-five years ago. It was obvious to me, as a busy obstetrician working in New York City and endeavoring to keep up with the latest research and methodology, that great advances were being made in my field. Obstetrics was becoming more of a science and, perhaps, less of an art. But I continued to observe that the distress of couples who lost a pregnancy or failed to conceive or hold a pregnancy after repeated IVF treatments was often underappreciated by medical professionals. No aspect of pregnancy had received as little attention as this "Cinderella" issue, which is so vitally important.

Reasons for the growing interest, both in the medical profession and among women themselves, include the increasing age of first-time mothers; the increasing numbers of infertile couples; the trend toward smaller families, so each conception becomes extremely important to the new parents; and the massive increase in cases of pregnancy as a result of IVF. When things go badly wrong, it hurts for women, and men, today to feel so out of control. The pain is not only emotional, but also physical, social, professional, and financial.

Moreover, society at large has no accepted ritual for couples who have suffered pregnancy loss. Often the grieving mother and father are sent home from the hospital empty-armed, only to feel the full extent of their loss when they are alone, isolated by their grief. They may have each other to lean on, but until recently there has been little sympathy forthcoming and few opportunities to deal with their grief even from family and friends, let alone professionals.

Doctors have been hampered by the lack of medical answers as to why miscarriages occurred. In the past they were also frustrated by the lack of information about the early stages of pregnancy—the first 12 weeks, known as the first trimester. This lack of knowledge resulted in either no treatment or inappropriate treatment, administered out of desperation to do something to maintain the pregnancy. Patients tended to go from doctor to doctor, having various tests done in a random fashion and without much coordination.

In my practice I have found that many of these couples want to talk and express feelings about their loss. They have found it difficult to grieve over something they could not visualize. Many also feel responsible for causing the miscarriage: guilt and self-blame are common emotions, although in the majority of cases the guilt is without foundation.

Eventually, I started a clinic at Mount Sinai Hospital, in New York City, where we treated women who had experienced recurrent miscarriage. The Pregnancy Support Clinic was staffed by physicians, nurses, and social workers. Besides the best we could offer in medical intervention, the women and their partners received emotional support, and a hotline was established so that patients could call whenever they felt anxious about certain symptoms.

Patients respond well to this rational, orderly approach to their problem. They also appreciate the reassurance offered by concerned professionals.

The good news resulting from the establishment of special clinics, plus further research and new technological developments, is that more and more causes of miscarriage are now being discovered and appropriate treatments offered. Significantly, the psychological consequences of miscarriage are being appreciated and studied. Couples can feel confident that their pregnancies are being managed by dedicated doctors, nurses, and social workers, and that if a miscarriage does happen, the same level of care will be put into action after a loss.

The message of *Preventing Miscarriage* is that doctors are now better prepared to investigate a miscarriage—in some cases, under special circumstances, even a first-time miscarriage. Women do not always have to undergo three or more losses before their problem is appreciated and treated.

There is a lot of hope within the pages of this book. The medical profession has a better understanding of the stress and anxiety that miscarriage can provoke, and there have been many advances in this area. Readers owe it to themselves, their families, and their doctors to become as wise as possible.

If you are reading this book, maybe you are still grieving for the loss of a child. I want to emphasize that both Carol Dix, my coauthor, and I are sensitive to your feelings, which is why we want to pass on to you some of the new optimism. Many of the women's stories that you will be reading in these pages tell of years of despair, feelings of failure, and disappointment to the point where they nearly gave up all hope. Then, thanks to new areas of investigation into the causes of miscarriage and to new treatments, they now have beautiful, normal, healthy babies in their nurseries at home.

Their stories are full of courage, fighting spirit, and determination to bring the reproductive cycle to its natural fruition. We hope that these stories, coupled with the most up-to-date research in an ever-changing world of medical information, will help boost your spirits, too. You will learn about the newest developments in the prevention of recurrent miscarriages, the results of which are only now being appreciated. For doctors, as well as for the couples involved, this is all very exciting.

Miscarriage need no longer be a soul-wrenching mystery to you and your partner. It need no longer remain a source of chronic depression, feelings of inadequacy or failure, or a bottomless pit of lonely pain. There really is hope and a strong direction for the future for most couples if you know what tests are available and how best to approach this difficult period of your family life.

—Jonathan Scher, M.D.

PART ONE

Miscarriage and You

⚘

1

✿

"You Don't Ever Forget a Miscarriage"

✿

I don't see how you can be expected to "forget" a miscarriage. Even if it happened at only 8 weeks, there had been a baby inside you. There was hope and planning and dreams. We don't let each other grieve the right way. It's not "just a miscarriage," but a *baby* that has been lost. Whether you know someone for 10 years, or it's a baby that's only been inside of you a few weeks, there's still a relationship there that you have made. It's become part of your life.

All the time, women like me hear that "It's God's way" or "It was meant to be." But those words don't take away the pain, even if they're right. If you want to talk about it at all, friends, relatives, they try and change the subject, and you'll be asked, "Do you want a cup of tea or coffee?" What I say is, If it was really God's will then why does He let me get pregnant so easily?

If a friend of yours died, people wouldn't say, "Oh, it was God's way," and if you're crying over that death, they wouldn't say, "Stop crying." I've found that the only people who really understand what I'm going through are others who've undergone miscarriages; they can share their sense of loss with you.

I was really strong for the first miscarriage. But by this third one, I've just been thrown. How strong can you be? I hold on for my husband's and my daughter's sakes. But I cry when I'm alone in the evenings. It's something I'll never forget.

❦

Debbie is not a wealthy woman. Her husband works as a store manager. They can barely afford the medical bills involved in fertility treatment. Yet her deep desire for another child drives her on. She is being treated for an autoimmune disorder that has been detected as the possible cause of her problem.

Philippa, socially Debbie's opposite, is the wife of a wealthy lawyer. A graciously attractive woman, she, too, had a daughter before suffering any problems with miscarriages. That daughter is now 11 years old; in the years since her birth Philippa has lost five more babies. Recently, Philippa experienced another devastating loss, a late miscarriage at 23 weeks. At the age of 42, both she and her husband feel that they have lost control over this vital area of their lives.

"No One Knows How to Respond to You"

✸

There are people for whom life always goes easily. Until I was 30, I was one of those people. Then, after that first miscarriage, I realized I had passed through a door onto the other side, a magic door. Now I'm with all those people who suffer, who grieve, who cannot make life run along the lines they'd prefer.

Once you've gone through that door, most people just don't know how to respond to you. I can't really blame them; until it happened to me I wouldn't have known, either. But I've had friends cross the street rather than have to confront me. Most people, I think, would prefer to pretend the baby never happened, rather than talk about your loss with you.

After the loss of this latest baby—a little girl, born at 23 weeks—my husband took me away for a vacation to Barbados. It was lucky we were staying at a very proper English resort, because the one thing I didn't want was anyone becoming too close and friendly. How do you answer the common question, "How many children do you have?" What I want to say to them is something along the lines of "I have one live child and a garden full of babies we have buried." But you can't do that to your random well-wisher, can you? I'm not strong enough yet to take such a stance.

On the way back from that vacation, the movie on the plane unexpectedly showed a scene of a woman giving birth. That was the last thing I wanted to see. But it was a jammed flight and I couldn't get out of my seat. I took the headphones off so I wouldn't have to listen. But I burst into tears. There I was still postmiscarriage, bleeding heavily, and my milk started to gush forth. I was wet and crying uncontrollably. The woman sitting next to me tried to move as far away as she could get. But the stewardess kindly brought me a blanket to cover myself.

You go through all the same hormonal and emotional changes as after a full-term birth. And you can't explain your situation to anyone. Would anyone have wanted to hear?

❧

For some women, the loss of a baby may be almost unnoticed. Happening in the very early weeks following conception, the blood loss often appears like a heavy but late period. To other women, the loss is traumatic, painful, and most deeply experienced. Today, the medical and caring professions are becoming aware that no woman should be ignored at the time of such loss. If the woman was emotionally involved with the pregnancy, then the miscarriage should be seen as an important time in her life, and in that of the couple. No one, neither the woman nor her partner, should be left rocking themselves to sleep at night, vexed with unanswered questions such as: Why did this happen to me? What is wrong with us that we cannot produce a baby? Why has such sadness been thrust upon us? Can we be sure it won't happen again? Could we possibly bear the pain of going through the excitement, and the hope, of another pregnancy only to suffer this devastating loss one more time?

An early miscarriage may be a normal, natural way for nature to abort a deformed or unhealthy embryo; or it may be a sign of some very real cause as to why some pregnancies will not hold and go to term. So let us now turn to some questions that are most often asked by women and their partners when they have miscarried.

What Is the Actual Definition of a Miscarriage?

The term *miscarriage* (which your doctor may also call a *spontaneous abortion*) actually refers to the loss of a pregnancy up to the end of week 20. This is now an accepted working definition in the medical literature. We used to define a miscarriage as the loss of a pregnancy before week 28 because, until recently, a fetus that was less than 28 weeks old could not be regarded as viable. Now, thanks to new developments in science and technology, we are able to save some babies born at 26 weeks. There have even been a few cases of younger babies surviving to normal life, so the cut-off point has been pushed back to 20 weeks.

That still leaves us with a twilight area for those women who lose babies between weeks 20 and 26—a time when fetal life may yet be saved—and their condition might even be termed *premature labor*. Major medical advances are being made in treating babies of this age. The causes for any loss between weeks 20 and 26 should still be investigated so that we can find out just what happened in order to prevent a recurrence.

Can the Baby's Weight Be a Definition?

There has been some discussion in the medical literature as to whether the baby's weight would provide a better definition. For example, could the lost embryo or fetus that weighs 500 grams or less be defined as a miscarriage? But this approach is faulty since at 20 weeks a baby may weigh 300, 500, or 600 grams. What is most important is how long the baby has been in the uterus and its level of physical development.

There is one documented case of an infant born two months

early, at a weight of 397 grams, who survived for at least a year. That means the baby was born at 32 weeks weighing just 1 pound instead of the expected 3 to 4 pounds. This baby was not in fact that premature at 32 weeks, but *growth-retarded*—a clear distinction—because the fetus was too low in weight for its age.

To use one other example, if you give birth to a 5½-pound baby at 36 weeks, that baby might suffer from lung disease. Ironically, if you smoked heavily or had high blood pressure and gave birth to a 5-pound baby at full term (40 weeks), the baby would have the better chance of survival simply because it would have been alive in the uterus longer and its organs would have developed further. So you can see that the weight of a baby alone does not always tell the full story.

Although many couples these days pray that premature labor around 24 to 26 weeks will indeed mean a live baby—one who can be nurtured and kept alive in a hospital's neonatal intensive care unit (NICU)—tragedy sometimes results from such a situation. In Chapter 10, we will return to the story of Philippa. She and her husband have run the gamut of experiences, including premature labor at 23 weeks with a baby born alive and, hopefully, capable of independent life. As Philippa describes so eloquently, the human cost, in emotional, financial, and spiritual terms, can be catastrophic.

Just How Often Do Miscarriages Happen?

Whether the statistic is 1 in 10 or 1 in 100,000, when it happens to *you* the incidence seems irrelevant. To you, it's 100 percent. Nevertheless, because we know so little about miscarriages and the real number of occurrences, most people ask this question.

The answer, unfortunately, is that no one knows for certain.

Every published scientific study and magazine article offers a different statistic, because the various studies tend to concentrate on different stages of miscarriage.

What we do know is that every day many more miscarriages happen than we record, because some may appear as just a heavy period. For example, women who use intrauterine devices, or IUDs, for contraception may be miscarrying when they are having a period. Also, women tend to tell their doctors about a prior miscarriage only when they are into their first ongoing pregnancy.

Of clinically diagnosed pregnancies, where the woman has missed a period and knows she is pregnant, about 15 to 25 percent will end in miscarriage. In fact, in a group of women aged 20 to 40, 1 in 4 stated she had had a miscarriage. An equal number of implanted embryos (known as *chemical pregnancies*), miscarry before the missed period, giving a total figure of 30 to 50 percent for all "implanting" embryos—the ones that have actually embedded in the uterus—that miscarry. About another 15 percent of fertilized eggs are lost before implantation, giving a total loss rate of 45 to 65 percent for all fertilized eggs.

Furthermore, 1 in 300 couples suffer three or more miscarriages back to back; this is the original definition of recurrent miscarriage. This means that about 200,000 women suffer two consecutive miscarriages and about 80,000 couples suffer three back-to-back miscarriages each year in the United States.

Advanced maternal age is a known cause of miscarriage, and this is influencing the statistics, since more women are having babies at a later age. But now we are beginning to get a better idea of just how common miscarriages really are, because pregnancy tests can diagnose conception 6 to 7 days after the egg and sperm meet, that is, 8 to 10 days before a woman would even notice a missed period. Together with the use of ultrasound from the earliest stages of pregnancy, the new forms of technology can be very accurate.

Indeed, both ultrasound and the use of very sensitive pregnancy tests have completely altered the practice of obstetrics. Thirty years ago, before a doctor could tell a woman she was definitely pregnant, she probably already knew herself! Tests in those days often did not yield results until the woman was 2 to 3 months pregnant. The patient's urine had to be injected into frogs or rabbits, which were then sacrificed and examined to diagnose pregnancy. Today, if every woman had a very early pregnancy test done *every month,* throughout her reproductive life, then the recorded rate of spontaneous miscarriage would probably turn out to be even higher.

The term *ultrasound* has become extremely familiar to any woman who has been pregnant. Many hospitals and doctors' offices now offer routine ultrasound scans, especially in the early weeks of pregnancy. Sonography makes use of high-frequency sound waves that cannot be heard by the human ear. They are emitted from a probe (transducer) attached to the ultrasound machine. As they pass through human tissue, they rebound at each surface, returning to the machine where an image is created. It is important to know that ultrasound has nothing to do with x-rays and is not a form of radiation.

With skilled usage, ultrasound has become a great boon to the obstetrician. Modern ultrasound equipment has all sorts of highly developed software that allows both you and your doctor to see very high resolution images. You will be able to see the hair on the baby's scalp; this would have been impossible a few years ago. And now there is even 3-D equipment that enables your doctor to detect certain structural changes in the baby's organs—for example, in the brain—as it gives such fine detail.

We can now estimate a baby's maturity accurately and can therefore double-check the mother's dates. In early pregnancy, between weeks 5 and 12, ultrasound predicts maturity within 3 to 5 days, which is an extraordinary rate of accuracy. If you have a scan in the first 8 to 9 weeks of your pregnancy to measure the length of the baby (known as the "crown-rump length") and a problem then arises later in the pregnancy, the doctor has an accurate baseline assessment of the baby's maturity. However, as pregnancy progresses, the dating becomes less accurate (and is quite inaccurate after 32 weeks).

So you see why it is so important that you begin to make regular visits to your doctor at the very earliest stage of a new pregnancy. Few pregnancies take place these days without the support of ultrasound, which is one of the biggest changes in the management and care of pregnancy in the past 30 years. It is safe and, with smaller machines, is usually performed in your doctor's office.

Ultrasound helps not only in the accuracy of dating and assessing the maturity of the baby, but it also means the doctor can watch the baby's growth progress by doing repeated scans if necessary. It is also extremely helpful as an adjunct to some of the more advanced tests, such as alpha-fetoprotein (AFP) testing, chorionic villus sampling (CVS), amniocentesis, and nuchal (neck) fold screening, for which accurate dates are vital.

Why Were Three Miscarriages Once Necessary Before Investigation Occurred?

The medical profession has always relied on the odds in favor of a couple having a normal, healthy pregnancy after a miscarriage as proof positive that miscarriages can be overcome naturally. This was the main reason for insisting that a woman have three consecutive miscarriages, with no live birth in between, before undertaking an investigation into the causes. Another reason for waiting, of course, was that little was known about the causes of a miscarriage until recently.

But the chances of having a live birth rapidly worsen after miscarriage.

- After one spontaneous abortion, the chances for a successful pregnancy next time are almost 87 percent (i.e., a 13 percent chance for a miscarriage).
- After two spontaneous abortions, the chances for a successful pregnancy are 60 percent (a 40 percent chance of miscarriage).
- After three or more spontaneous abortions, the chances for giving birth are 40 percent (a 60 percent chance of miscarriage).
- After a fifth miscarriage, there is over 90 percent chance of miscarrying again.

These figures suggest that some recurrent or persistent medical cause may be operating, and without investigation of the cause and further treatment, another pregnancy may be lost.

Why Has Information on Miscarriage Been So Slow in Coming?

No aspect of pregnancy has received as little attention as the first trimester of pregnancy. Yet by week 12, the embryo has formed most of its organs; hence, this is known as the period of organogenesis. This is the most likely time for a miscarriage. From an ethical point of view, it is a very difficult time to investigate a pregnancy in the first trimester, since no tests can be performed that at this critical stage of life may harm the embryo. And certainly there is little place for the usual scientific method—the double-blind trial, whereby some women are given a treatment that is thought to be effective, while a control group is not—as this may lead to withholding necessary treatment.

The earlier lack of interest in the first trimester has kept our statistics uncertain and our scientific knowledge meager. In fact, even standard texts included very little on the subject. Until recently, moreover, women who miscarried in the first few weeks of pregnancy were regarded as gynecologic problems rather than as patients trying to have a baby. Fortunately, however, the situation regarding miscarriages is now changing.

Waiting Until Three Miscarriages Have Occurred Is Not Always Necessary

Any miscarriage is tragic. No matter how many miscarriages you have had and no matter how early in the pregnancy they occurred, they are still emotionally devastating. Well-meaning expressions of sympathy such as "Don't worry, you can try again" or "It wasn't really a baby" are now generally acknowledged to be the wrong approach to take.

Mothers undergo huge hormonal fluctuations, and we tend to think these grow along with her swelling belly. The major changes in a pregnant woman's hormonal makeup take place early in pregnancy, almost immediately after conception. So when you lose a desired pregnancy, it feels almost like you have lost a child, an anticipated child. There is scientific (i.e., hormonal) proof that these feelings occur. At last women are being believed.

Now that we can diagnose most causes of miscarriage and treatment is available in the majority of cases, it seems kinder to investigate women after two miscarriages, and maybe even one, rather than make them suffer through three such experiences. The success factor is increasing all the time as medical knowledge improves. One of the big breakthroughs has been in the field of reproductive immunology, which I will explain more fully in Chapter 8.

There are other reasons why each pregnancy should now be viewed as premium:

- People are tending to have smaller and smaller families.
- Women are delaying childbearing until a certain point in their careers.
- It just does not make emotional, or even economic, sense to allow what is coldly termed "pregnancy wastage" to continue.
- With each miscarriage, the chances of another increase, and so does the likelihood of a causative factor.
- If a woman is 35 years of age or older, and this is her first pregnancy loss—especially if it was proven to be genetically normal—it would be a pity not to search for a cause of the miscarriage and possibly to treat the problem. Some of the tests are simple to do and don't involve elaborate medical intervention.
- Assisted reproduction technologies (ART) such as IVF, are physically, emotionally, and financially taxing, and women are devastated if they miscarry. It is important to determine why they have miscarried before they undergo another treatment.

"It's One Heck of a Way to Be Pregnant!"

Robert and Grace went through both in vitro fertilization and immunological treatment against miscarriage before giving birth to their son, who is now a beautiful 9-month-old. They have a very down-to-earth approach to the problem that dogged their lives for so many years. As Robert says:

❧

When you suffer a miscarriage, or infertility, you become part of a growing underground, a subgroup of people all in the same situation, and you feel no one out there is addressing your problems. It's an extraordinarily stressful time that might go on for years. In a day and age when people are used to feeling in control of their lives, it hurts to feel so totally out of control.

Even when you do manage to get pregnant again, you daren't tell your friends or family. There's none of the normal glow and enjoyment of pregnancy. It's a very strange panicky time, very secretive. And for the man, the extra stress is in feeling he has to be emotionally tough to carry his wife's total vulnerability.

It's one heck of a way to be pregnant!

❧

What Should You Expect from Your Doctor After a Miscarriage?

Once you and your partner have had time to overcome your grief and feel ready to approach another conception, then it is time to consult an obstetrician about your future.

Your doctor will ask not only about the bleeding or cramping that led up to the miscarriage but also about your previous general medical and menstrual history. There will be many questions. Each question and answer may suggest its own line of treatment. For example, did you have late onset of menarche (the age of your first period) or a history of missed periods, either of which might be a sign of poor ovulation? If so, you may need an *endometrial biopsy* to test for hormonal problems. If you have a history of severe pain with your periods *(dysmenorrhea)*, it might also lead your doctor to look for an abnormality in the shape of your uterus or *endometriosis*, which is now considered to be an autoimmune disorder and can be treated medically. If you have had more than one miscarriage, is there a pattern that has emerged? If they were all in the second trimester, for example, the entrance to the uterus may be too weak to hold a pregnancy. This is called an *incompetent cervix.*

You will probably be asked about activity levels of all kinds—whether, for example, you partake in very vigorous sports. If you have been very active, you may be advised to rest more during the next pregnancy, at least until you are past the first 12 to 13 weeks, or beyond the point where you last miscarried. Similarly, you might be advised to avoid sexual intercourse, at least until the end of the first trimester.

Is there a family history of miscarriage on either your or your partner's side? This might suggest a familial problem. If your mother had numerous miscarriages, maybe she was given diethylstilbestrol (DES) when she was pregnant with you, which may cause you to have fertility problems or to miscarry. DES use was discontinued in 1972, so it does not apply if you were born after that period.

Do you or your partner take drugs? Both medications and recreational drugs can be factors in causing miscarriages. Do either of you smoke or drink heavily?

As you can see, your partner's history is also relevant, and he should go to the doctor with you, at least during your first consultation.

Your medical history may include details of induced abortions by means of a D&C (dilation and curettage), especially if these procedures were done some years ago, when the entrance to the uterus was probably opened mechanically with metal dilators.

There is an increase in second-trimester (13 to 26 weeks) miscarriages in women with a previous history of multiple terminated pregnancies—multiple being as many as six or seven—most likely because of an incompetent cervix, a result of stretching during the repeated abortions. Much of the data on the effect of repeated terminations on miscarriage has come from Eastern Europe, where abortion has long been used as a form of contraception. But be reassured: a history of two or three early-induced abortions (terminations) should not increase your risk of a miscarriage. Nevertheless, you must tell your doctor about any abortion history.

After all the questions, the doctor's physical examination usually includes a general physical checkup to detect any medical disorders and a pelvic examination to see if your pelvic organs are healthy and the shape of your uterus is normal. When the routine Pap smear is done, your doctor may take a sample of your cervical secretion and culture it to detect infections that, although they may be asymptomatic, could contribute to a miscarriage.

The doctor may then discuss with you and your partner the various possibilities that may have resulted in your problem, and a series of tests may be planned depending on your particular case.

The possible causes of a miscarriage—and tests to be done—are listed below. They will be explained in more detail later in the book.

1. *Genetics.* If a genetic cause is suspected, you and your partner will probably be referred to a genetics testing center. There you will be interviewed and blood will be drawn from both of you for chromosome testing. White cells from both blood samples are grown to see if

you and your partner have abnormal chromosomes, which may give a clue as to why you are miscarrying. If they are not normal, however, this is not necessarily predictive for a future miscarriage.

2. *Anatomic or uterine abnormalities.* If, from your history, this seems to be the cause of your miscarriage, you will be referred to a radiologist for a hysterogram to see if the uterus is normal in structure and to check for cervical incompetence—that is, to see if the cervix is too weak to hold a pregnancy. Antibiotics are often given before this procedure to prevent uterine infection from the injection of the dye. A hysterogram is an x-ray, usually done in a radiologist's office. It may cause some cramping and mild discomfort since the dye is injected into the uterus through the cervix.

There is another excellent way to test to see if you have enough room in the uterus: a saline sonogram (or ultrasound), which does not involve an x-ray and can be done in your doctor's office or by a radiologist. Before the transvaginal probe is inserted into the vagina, a small amount of saline solution is injected through the cervix into the uterine cavity; this makes the uterus open up to reveal any abnormalities.

Another new technique is known as *hysteroscopy,* which involves the doctor looking into the uterine cavity with a special telescope, or *hysteroscope.* This is normally done under general anesthetic or with heavy sedation as it can cause a lot of discomfort.

3. *Endocrine (hormonal) disorders.* Your checkup may have given a clue as to some endocrine, or hormonal, cause. The doctor may order blood to be drawn to study levels of thyroid hormone in the body, as thy-

roid disturbances may contribute to a miscarriage. Also, in order to ensure that during your menstrual cycle you produce enough progesterone—the most important hormone in early pregnancy—the doctor may order a blood progesterone measurement in the second half of your next cycle. You may also be asked to keep a temperature chart. The rise in your temperature at the time of egg production, or ovulation—known as the thermal shift—indicates an adequate amount of progesterone. Ovulation occurs approximately 14 days before a period.

The endometrial biopsy is a method of determining if you are ovulating at the correct stage for fertilization (synchronous fertilization) and if you are producing an adequate supply of hormones after ovulation to maintain a pregnancy. It involves taking a sample of your uterine lining, late in the menstrual cycle (days 21 to 24 from the start of your period, known as the "window of implantation"). The procedure does cause some short-lived cramping, for which a mild painkiller may be taken. How the biopsy is done will be explained in Chapter 5.

Another hormone that doctors often monitor following a miscarriage is prolactin. If this runs at a very high level, it can interfere with early pregnancy, but treatment is available.

Polycystic ovarian syndrome (PCOS) and diabetes are other hormone disorders routinely tested for. PCOS is common in young women. Symptoms of this hormonal disorder include irregular or missed periods, and sometimes excess weight and acne. It is a cause of infertility and because it is linked to a harmful antibody, or cytokine, it may also lead to miscarriage. However, it can be remedied, if diagnosed.

4. *Infections.* To detect these, samples of secretions are taken from the vagina and the cervix, very much like a Pap smear. Your partner must also be tested to exclude infection. His samples are taken from a sterile collection of seminal fluid (which may be done as part of a semen analysis) and sent to the laboratory for culture. Alternatively, it can be done in the doctor's office by passing a fine sterile Q-tip into his urethra at the tip of his penis. However, most men balk at this!

5. *Medical disorders.* If, at the time of your examination, you are discovered to be suffering from a medical disorder such as uncontrolled diabetes, thyroid disease, heart disease, or high blood pressure, you will be referred to your internist for treatment. It is known that general medical disorders may contribute to miscarriages.

There are hereditary factors that cause blood clotting which are now seen to be an important cause of miscarriage or infertility. Known as *thrombophilias*, you should be tested for these in your blood, especially if you have a strong family history of heart attacks, high blood pressure, or strokes, as treatment is available.

6. *Placental abnormalities.* It is now becoming extremely important to test pregnancy loss tissue—even from previous miscarriages—to see whether these might have been caused by certain abnormalities in the placenta. This tissue is the junction between you and your pregnancy. Your doctor should send the tissue to a placental pathologist. In the United States pathological tissue samples are kept for over 20 years, so the tissue slides from any previous miscarriages should be avail-

able for examination. This information may also help with the treatment plan for your next pregnancy. For example, was there a clotting problem or an infection or was it likely an immune or chromosomal problem?

7. *Mind-body medicine and the role of stress.* I will talk more about this important aspect of miscarriage later in the book. We now have evidence that stress may affect the mother's hormonal and immune systems, so relieving stress should have a beneficial effect on your pregnancy.

8. *Environmental causes.* Although there is little we can do to counter the effects of acid rain and ground pollution, there are things we can control in our lives. Pregnant women should avoid the harmful effects of smoking (including secondhand smoke) and alcohol.

9. *Immune disorders.* Immunology is the study of the body's response when it encounters something foreign. The immunological paradox of pregnancy, discussed in the Introduction, is an exciting avenue of research. Scientists are trying to discover why the embryo, which includes the father's "foreign" tissue, is not rejected by the mother's body. In other circumstances, the woman's body would normally produce antibodies to reject this half-foreign embryo. However, it is now known that the antibodies in pregnancy can also become protective and turn into a different type of antibody, allowing the embryo to grow for as long as 40 weeks in the woman's body.

As mentioned earlier, this is known as the *immunologic paradox of pregnancy.* It is the only example in mammalian nature that a foreign substance is allowed to grow in the body for that length of time. Just think

what happens to germs, skin grafts, and organ transplants. Our body works at rejecting these foreign
invaders. Pregnancy is therefore a remarkable and awe-
inspiring event.

If acceptance of the embryo doesn't take place, the
pregnancy fails. In this case the woman's blood should
be screened for a possible *allo-immune disorder*. Allo-
immune means reacting to something introduced from
outside the body. Allo-immune disoders are asymptomatic, so they should not affect the woman at any time
other than pregnancy.

The woman's blood should also be tested for *auto-
antibodies* (antibodies that attack one's own tissue).
These are important factors in recurrent miscarriage.
Antiphospholipid antibodies (APAs) account for many
miscarriages that were previously thought to be inexpli-
cable. Testing for them is now an accepted investigation for a woman who miscarries. Seven different APAs
have been identified thus far. The best known is the *anticardiolipin antibody*. A similar type of antibody is *lupus anticoagulant*. Successful treatments are available
for these varieties.

The woman's blood should be tested for two other
types of auto-antibodies: *antithyroid antibodies,* which
may be present even if thyroid function tests are normal; and *antinuclear antibodies*, which attack the cell
nucleus and are found in autoimmune diseases such as
systemic lupus erythematosus (SLE). Both types of antibody can cause miscarriages and lead to IVF failure.

It is especially important to test for levels of immune Natural Killer (NK) cells, which can cause miscarriage and failed IVF if levels are elevated.

Also from the blood sample, the woman's *platelets* (blood factors important in clotting) can be measured to ensure that levels are normal; platelet levels sometimes fall in immune disorders.

10. *Sperm DNA Integrity Testing.* This is a test to see if there are any abnormalities in the protein makeup of the father's sperm that may cause decreased fertility or miscarriage.

When Can You Try to Conceive Again Following a Miscarriage?

The decision to start a new pregnancy lies solely with you as a couple. There used to be conflicting advice about whether to wait one month, three months, or even longer. It has now been shown that there is no medical reason for waiting—other than to make sure you are emotionally and psychologically ready to begin again—unless of course you are undergoing treatment for a specific cause of your miscarriage.

In saying that you should give yourself a chance to recover psychologically, I am also referring to the hormonal changes your body has undergone. For example, it takes one to two months for all the pregnancy hormones to leave your bloodstream, which means that even three or four weeks after a complete miscarriage or a D&C, you could still have a positive pregnancy test! Usually your period returns four to six weeks after a miscarriage, and you could begin trying to conceive during that cycle if you wish. You do not have to wait. Indeed, it has been shown that a pregnancy conceived soon after a miscarriage is at no greater risk of miscarrying.

People's emotional reactions to miscarriages vary enormously.

For some, part of the reaction evolves from fear, because miscarriages tend to happen so suddenly, with pain, bleeding, and maybe some loss of tissue. There's the rush to the hospital, the mystery surrounding the cause, the grief, and the feeling that maybe somehow you were to blame. Fear grows into anxiety because of all the unanswered questions.

What If No Cause Is Found?

If, even after intensive investigations by your doctor, no cause for your miscarriage has been found, there are still certain precautions you can take. I would recommend that during your next pregnancy you take it very easy, with as much rest, even occasionally bed rest, as possible in the first 9 to 10 weeks.

Once you have seen the fetal heartbeat on the sonogram, at weeks 6 to 7, your anxiety should decrease significantly. This will help give the pregnancy the optimal chance of continuing normally.

Keeping a Positive Attitude

When you're pregnant once again, it's important to try to maintain a positive attitude and not dwell on the possibility of another miscarriage. I know this can be an almost impossible task, especially when you come to the dreaded day or week of the previous loss. But stress and emotional anxiety may play some part in future miscarriages. If you experience a lot of chronic fear, I would recommend asking your doctor for a referral to a therapist or a social worker to help you deal with those feelings. The previous miscarriage may have resulted in excessive guilt feelings or caused problems between you and your husband. Relieving stress will make you feel more comfortable during testing and in the new pregnancy.

Finding Your Way to a Normal Pregnancy

If your doctor is monitoring your pregnancy hormone levels and checking up on the pregnancy with regular ultrasound scans, and if you make it past the sometimes tricky period between weeks 9 and 13, by which stage the placenta is fully developed, you can slowly resume more normal activities. When you see the first fetal movements on a sonogram, around week 8, this is an excellent sign that the pregnancy will progress safely and you are unlikely to miscarry. Your doctor will continue to see you often to ensure that all continues to go well.

"How Do You Find the Strength to Go On?"

This is the remarkable story of Megan. Now 42, with a 2½-year-old daughter, Megan is a book editor, contemplative and certainly wise to the problems that can beset a pregnancy. Her first pregnancy had been at the age of 32. She doesn't think she was really putting off having a child; rather, she had experienced some major stress in her work and from both parents dying of cancer.

❦

When you have a child at nearly 40, you've done a lot beforehand. You've socialized, held down a career, so you're prepared to give your all to this pregnancy. The devastation of fearing you'll lose the baby late in pregnancy is unbearable. By then the baby has become a person to you. So for me to go through ultimate bed rest for several months was no great hardship. It's like being in a war zone; I was doing it to protect my child from imminent danger.

There I was in my early thirties and no one knew what was wrong with me. It appeared that I was having a breakdown, with all the stresses going on around me. In fact, I had an ectopic pregnancy. It was terminated with a chemotherapy drug. The whole experience was very sad and made more so as that was an anticancer drug. I also knew I'd had a poor fallopian tube. But I became pregnant again four years later. I was immediately given a sonogram to rule out another ectopic pregnancy. The doctor at the time felt I should find a specialist in high-risk pregnancy, as they discovered fibroids. It was rather a scary start, but everything seemed to be fine until the 23rd week. I had a routine appointment, where I was found to be dilated to the degree that the amniotic sac was bulging through the cervix.

Looking back, I suppose the pregnancy was over there and then, but everyone tried to keep it going. The doctor kept me lying flat on my back, but no one mentioned putting in a stitch [cerclage] to keep the cervix closed. I was in the hospital for two days, when they discovered an infection. They induced delivery, knowing the baby would die. So I had to go through delivery of a dead baby. After that, I felt very determined to get pregnant again and also to find out what had happened. The pathology report came back with cause of death as "infection," which goes with a dilated cervix.

By then, I'd begun researching and reading about pregnancy, and I could see there was a debate as to whether the opening cervix leads to infection, or was it the other way around? I read a lot online about the significance of vaginal infections and joined bulletin boards of other women who have undergone pregnancy loss. I also decided in a future pregnancy I would need a stitch. By this point, I had also read Dr. Scher's book and his section on incompetent cervix. I made an appointment to see him and was reassured by his views on how to manage a problem cervix.

I was very lucky because I got pregnant again in under a year (aware that the years were now ticking by and by now I was 39). At first, I felt panicky. I had to have a sonogram to ensure it wasn't ectopic. I was put on heparin injections, baby aspirin, and progesterone suppositories. There were also regular early-pregnancy hormone tests. Cerclage was planned for 13 to 14 weeks, but the cervix began to soften and I was sent for an earlier stitch. Because of my age I first had the nuchal-fold sonogram test to narrow down the likelihood of chromosome problem.

So the stitch was put in by 12 weeks. It gave me a lot of confidence and I was happy as I felt that they were taking such good care of me. It was inserted under epidural anesthesia, and after that I went onto partial bed rest. I have to admit to feeling confused just what "partial" meant. Should it be half a day or a couple of hours? I was constantly worried that I might be doing something wrong. Also, it's obviously not an exact science, so there are no definite rules to go by. Fortunately, because of my work situation, as an editor, I could do a lot of work at home on the sofa with a frame holding the book.

Until the end of the 5th month, things seemed to be progressing fine. Then, when I went in for a routine appointment, they discovered that the cervix had funneled a lot and the amniotic fluid sac was pressing on the stitch. I was admitted into the hospital, flat on my back. I never got up again until the baby was born! I was so afraid that, even to go for a sonogram, I would not lift myself up. They had to carry me flat onto a stretcher. Of course, I'd do deep breathing and leg exercises to prevent a blood clot from forming.

How can you survive four months of bed rest? Well, the computer, Internet, and e-mail have changed things a lot. I'd divide my day up, working in the mornings, and in the afternoons I taught myself Russian. I just took the most conservative approach. My legs were elevated nearly the whole time. Every evening, my husband would come to visit, poor man. A couple of faithful friends came by. My office sent me work and helped keep me involved, as I had some long-term projects to work on.

As a high-risk pregnancy, you are on a fetal monitor all the time. They monitor you 24 hours a day, so I was constantly checking on this baby—which is why it becomes so real to you as a person. You're also very aware of the likelihood of an early delivery and a premature baby in intensive care. So, when the 25th week goes by, you've passed a milestone. Then the 28th week. The doctors take care of you on rotation. A doctor comes and talks to you every day, so everyone seems focused on you, all of which is so supportive. The nurses were wonderful. Because I was on the regular delivery unit, I knew all the staff, whereas other mothers only stayed a couple of days. You're like part of the family. The most amazing thing, too, is that it was all covered by insurance. For that I also have to give thanks.

Finally, by the 8th month, I was sent home. I was still so nervous that I determined to continue the complete bed rest, though I was told it could be partial. My husband would set up lunch for me in a cooler. It was the time of the 2000 elec-

tions, so I found a lot on TV to watch. I was on home monitoring then, which is expensive. You have a machine that
checks for uterine contractions and the baby's movements. It's
connected to the telephone, which is monitored by an agency.
By the end of that month, I was allowed up, as the baby was
big enough to be born. The stitch was taken out. I toddled
around, hardly daring to go outside. In the end, I went four
days overdue, maybe because some scarring held the cervix. I
had a forceps delivery, but I avoided a C-section.

And there she was—perfectly healthy and fine. I could
hardly believe it. Having gone through so much to keep this
pregnancy, I think it intensifies the pleasure of motherhood.
When you have a child at nearly 40, you've done plenty in the
world so you don't mind giving up some of your freedom.
Maybe bed rest is easier for someone like me, as I'm quite a
reader and an intellectual. But because of the devastation of
losing a baby late in pregnancy, when you can feel the person
who is there, it is so intense. It's like being in a war zone;
you're protecting this child from imminent danger. I'd do it
again—even knowing what it was like to spend those months
flat on my back.

ϒ

2

✢

When the Bleeding and Cramping Spell Trouble

Y ou're a normal, healthy woman, happily looking forward to
having a baby. Just like Megan, whose story appears in
Chapter 1, you're unlikely even to have thought about losing the
baby—unless a history of miscarriages has already dogged you or
a close relative—when suddenly events overtake your dreams.
You are thrown into an incomprehensible and strange underground world of tears and heartache.

The most common symptoms of an impending miscarriage
are bleeding and cramping. Yet bleeding in pregnancy is also very
commonplace and, in those who don't miscarry, may be quite
normal. So obviously, some distinction must be made between
what is normal and what may mean a possible miscarriage.

Up to 70 percent of pregnant women experience a degree of
blood loss during the early weeks of their pregnancy. How can

this happen when the blood flow of normal periods has ended? One reason is that until the 20th week of pregnancy, the uterine cavity is not entirely filled by the fetus and placenta, and as at all times in a woman's life, your hormone levels may still be fluctuating to some degree. Just as hormonal changes in the nonpregnant state lead to menstruation, so hormonal fluctuations in pregnancy can now lead to some staining. The bleeding is not coming from the embryo or fetus itself, but from the still-unoccupied uterine lining, and it in no way presents a danger to the developing life.

This type of bleeding, or staining, tends to occur especially at those times when you would normally be expecting a period had you not been pregnant, and usually around weeks 10 to 12, when the placenta takes over hormonal support of the pregnancy from the corpus luteum in the ovary. Or bleeding may occur when the fertilized embryo implants in the uterus, after its journey down the fallopian tube. A little spotting at this stage is not unusual.

If the staining is dark brown, it usually indicates that there is a very small amount of slow bleeding, which has been stagnant for a while. It is not fresh red blood, which would indicate more vigorous bleeding, and therefore is not a cause for panic. But if the bleeding becomes fresh and heavy, like a period or worse, or if there is cramping or severe backache, then there may be a real problem, and you should get into bed and contact your doctor.

As far as cramping is concerned, bear in mind that the uterus contracts at all times whether you are pregnant or not: during a period, during orgasm, and even at times in the normal course of a day. If you have miscarried before and feel some cramping, you are bound to become agitated. But it is often normal to cramp *without* bleeding during pregnancy.

I have found that women who have miscarried before can become so tense over the sensation of cramping that they may trigger a chain reaction known as spastic colon (or irritable bowel), which is caused by stimulation of the autonomic nervous system. This is the part of the nervous system that controls our internal organs. Through this type of nervous response, the colon, or large intestine, distends and fills with gas. The ensuing cramping is from the bowel, not the uterus, and is felt all over the stomach and not just at the location of the uterus. Your stomach will also be distended with gas. Extremely severe cramping, however, needs immediate investigation, as it may be an indication of an impending miscarriage or even a tubal (ectopic) pregnancy.

Bleeding is by far the most common sign of a threatened or inevitable miscarriage. Before I explain the various terms you are likely to hear from your doctor or the hospital staff for the different types of miscarriage, I want first to explain the best course of action to take if any symptoms occur.

What to Do When You Fear
You May Be Miscarrying

I am aware that panic is a commonly experienced emotion when things begin to go wrong, especially if you have miscarried previously. But panic, agitation, and aggravated distress, unfortunately, will only worsen the situation, so try to remain calm. This is my best advice: First, get to bed. If the cramps feel like real pain, lie on your side. If the pain is such that you feel the need to use painkillers, then that would be a sign to contact your doctor.

You don't necessarily have to call your doctor immediately if there is blood loss. But do call if the bleeding becomes a moderate flow (more than staining).

You might, quite naturally, be terrified that a miscarriage will lead to severe hemorrhage (which is, in fact, a synonym for heavy bleeding), ultimately even requiring a blood transfusion. But despite alarming stories that you may have heard over the years, even severe blood loss can be controlled by your doctor.

If the pregnancy is in its very early stages, that is, in the first 6 weeks, there is little chance of your bleeding so heavily that it becomes dangerous for you. You may have cramps and find that you pass a few clots. It may also be possible, if the pregnancy is still under 6 weeks, to avoid a dilatation and curettage if you miscarry. This is important to bear in mind, because repeated D&Cs may increase your risk of developing either adhesions (scarring) inside the uterus or an incompetent cervix, as Megan so vividly described. But you must rely on your doctor's advice.

If you are more than 7 weeks pregnant, then there may be heavy bleeding that can last for several hours. *You should contact your doctor*. Also, do not use tampons, only sanitary napkins. Make a note of how many you have used and how soaked they were; even collect all your pads and take them to show the doctor. It may not be possible to tell with accuracy from the amount of your bleeding whether you have lost the baby or not. But as a general rule, any bleeding that is heavier than a normal period is not a good sign.

Should You Have an Internal Examination If You Are Bleeding in Early Pregnancy?

Your doctor will probably want to perform a vaginal examination to check on the state of your cervix. He will need to know if your cervix is shortening or opening or if fetal tissue is already being expelled into the cervix or vagina. These are signs of inevitable miscarriage—one that *will* definitely occur—and there is usually no way in such cases to save the pregnancy and prevent the fetus from being expelled.

But if your cervix remains closed, then you may not have lost the baby. An ultrasound scan can help to show both you and your doctor the exact status of the pregnancy. Ideally, you will even be able to see the fetal heartbeat, which is the best of all circumstances.

If you have miscarried before, you may well worry either that the internal examination will increase the risk of further bleeding or that it will cause the threatened miscarriage to become an inevitable one. You can discuss this with your doctor. But it is unlikely that an internal examination would set off any miscarriage that was not already going to occur; and remember, the internal examination will provide your doctor with valuable information.

I mentioned in the previous chapter the enormous boon that ultrasound has been to the obstetrician, and nowhere is this more evident than in our treatment of a woman who has bled in early pregnancy. By using ultrasound to see a heartbeat, we can now diagnose whether fetal *life* is still present, even after heavy bleeding, and we can know with certainty whether you still have a good chance of continuing your pregnancy and producing a healthy baby. Before the introduction of ultrasound into obstetrics (in the early 1970s), there was no immediate way of knowing if the baby was still alive, and treatment was difficult to decide upon.

Your doctor may also test to see if your blood hormone levels are adequate, though it may take a day or two to get the results. Hormone values are less predictable than sonography because they may continue to be at normal levels even when the fetus is no longer alive. A regular pregnancy test would be of no value in determining whether the fetus is still alive, because it can read positive up to three weeks after a fetal death or a D&C. Human chorionic gonadotropin (HCG) is the hormone measured in a pregnancy test, and it can take up to 23 days to disappear from the blood system after an early pregnancy loss.

What If You Cannot See
the Fetal Heartbeat on the Sonogram?

If you are less than 7 to 8 weeks pregnant when you experience bleeding, the ultrasound scan may not be able to show a fetal heartbeat. (A *transvaginal* ultrasound probe can, however, show a heartbeat by 5 to 6 weeks.) You will be advised to return for another scan later, that is, beyond 8 weeks, to make sure the baby is still alive. If at week 8 or 9 there is still no sign of a fetal heart, it means the pregnancy has not survived. *Should your doctor at any time have doubts about the viability of the pregnancy, it is best to be patient and do nothing at the time, but rather to wait and repeat the scan in a few days' time. After all, your dates may be wrong and you may not be as far along in the pregnancy as you believed.*

Once you have been able to see for yourself that your baby's heart is beating, your anxieties should be allayed immediately. In itself, this quick reassurance seems to help the pregnancy proceed more smoothly. Ultrasound scans may be repeated as often as necessary, even every one to two weeks if there are any suspicions, so that both doctor and mother can be reassured. Indeed, I would say that if you have experienced any bleeding in early pregnancy, the use of ultrasound either abdominally or transvaginally could be a major component in determining the well-being of your pregnancy. It has made a big difference in managing bleeding in early pregnancy.

Is Ultrasound Safe in Early Pregnancy?

Ultrasound plays a major role in the management of normal pregnancy and is invaluable when complications such as bleeding or cramping occur. Because it is a high-frequency sound wave, out of range of the human ear, and not a form of ionizing radiation such as is used in x-rays, it is very safe. On the end of the transducer—the ultrasound probe placed either over the abdomen (abdominal probe) or in the vagina (transvaginal probe)—are metal plates or crystals that vibrate in response to an electrical current and send out sound waves, which are then reflected by your tissues according to their differing thickness, or density. A computer in the machine uses this data to create an image on the screen, enabling the doctor and the mother to "see" into the uterus and look at the fetus.

Abdominal ultrasound is useful only in pregnancies that have progressed beyond 6 to 8 weeks. The mother drinks enough water to fill her bladder, then gel is placed on her lower abdomen, and the probe is passed over her abdomen so that the ultrasound wave can create an image of the pregnant uterus. The transvaginal probe, a fairly recent improvement, is covered with a lubricated sheath and introduced into the vagina, then placed against the uterus, fallopian tubes, and ovaries. The state of the pregnancy can be examined and the fetal heart can be seen very early in the pregnancy—from at least weeks 5 or 6. This, of course, is a major advantage. Like the abdominal probe, the vaginal probe is safe to use in pregnancy. The transducer causes little or no discomfort at all.

Ultrasound also helps make intrauterine procedures, carried out in pregnancy, much safer: for example, it facilitates placement of the needle when we do an amniocentesis or chorionic villus sampling (CVS), and during extraction of blood from the umbilical cord for special tests.

An ectopic (tubal) pregnancy is potentially a very serious condition that may cause bleeding in early pregnancy. It can be diagnosed early by using ultrasound. This also means that the mother's health can be ensured and, through medical treatment with drugs, she can avoid the necessity of surgery to remove an ectopic pregnancy.

Both abdominal and transvaginal equipment take only minutes to use and give a wealth of information in early pregnancy. No harm has ever been done either to the fetus or to the mother from ultrasound.

If the Pregnancy Is Viable, What Should You Do Next?

Providing the cervix is closed and you have seen the live fetus on the sonogram, your doctor will probably tell you to go home and get as much rest as you can until the bleeding has ceased altogether. Try not to feel guilty. You should reassure yourself that nothing you have done caused the bleeding: your daily activities are not a factor in causing miscarriages. But adequate rest may be helpful in stopping the bleeding. Sedatives are not given as they do not help and may even be harmful to the fetus.

As you will read in several stories in this book, many women have successfully carried a pregnancy to term with the support of natural progesterone in the first trimester. If your doctor knows that prior to becoming pregnant you showed a *luteal phase deficiency* (LPD), also known as a *corpus luteum deficiency* (CLD), or if a blood test showed a very low level of progesterone, you may be a candidate for treatment with the natural hormone progesterone. It will be for your doctor to decide—unless you have strong objections to their use—whether progesterone suppositories or injections will help tide you over during this time of low progesterone levels or in the tricky period when the placenta takes over from the corpus luteum, at about weeks 9 to 11.

What Is So Special About Bed Rest?
Some Doctors Say It Is an Old Wives' Tale

Strangely, for something so utterly natural as relaxing and putting your feet up, there is wild controversy about bed rest within the medical profession. I believe in bed rest's value in pregnancy for many reasons. As you read in Megan's story, she remained in bed for much of the pregnancy. A friend of mine who is an eminent European obstetrician also believes strongly in the value of bed rest. One of his patients (a well-known film star) had suffered recurrent miscarriages for which no cause could be found. He treated her successfully just by keeping her in bed throughout the pregnancy. Of course, her husband built her a special hospital in which to spend her time!

You might read articles saying there is no scientific evidence to support the theory that bed rest is of value in preventing miscarriage or bleeding in pregnancy. The opposing attitude, in fact, is that it does not matter whether you hang curtains or go to the office or stay in bed; the outcome of the pregnancy will not be affected. I just happen to believe it does make a difference. And the evidence from my patients, even though it is anecdotal, seems to support this view.

Certainly, the value of bed rest in these high-risk pregnancies is difficult to prove scientifically. To do so, many women would have to agree to be part of a research study whereby they would retire to their beds for the whole of their pregnancies in special metabolic rooms. There, we could measure stress hormones and conduct other tests on the fetus to show whether bed rest helps in the pregnancy or not. Some in the study would have to be women who have never miscarried, and others would need to be women who had had recurrent miscarriages. Obviously this would be impossible practically. There are, however, published studies show-ing that women who work over a certain number of hours (in a variety of professions such as law and nursing) show greatly in-creased stress levels, which may lead to pregnancy complications, including miscarriage and infertility. There is also research show-ing that if animals are highly stressed, they produce excess harm-ful immune changes that may result in miscarriage. Some very new research has shown this may be the case in humans, too.

We suspect, moreover, that something very traumatic—such as loss of a job, being assaulted, or the death of a close relative—could trigger a miscarriage. Such a shock could cause unfavorable, hormonal, or immune responses, which may be a factor leading to the miscarriage.

But my major argument in support of bed rest is that nature planned it this way. It's our modern sophisticated minds that have tried to override nature's dictates. In the first trimester, the hor-monal balance of normal early pregnancy makes a woman very sleepy, fatigued, unable often to deal with the pressures of her work. Most women give up their exercise regimes at this time be-cause they are feeling nauseated and overly tired. Many lose their sexual desire (libido). All these energy levels usually return during a healthy pregnancy after week 10 to 12 (midtrimester), when the placenta has safely moved into action.

I think it's best to mimic nature to the degree possible. Why, we should ask ourselves, does nature make things happen this way? Although little has been proven to support my theory, it is likely that the corpus luteum—a tiny cyst formed after ovulation in the ovary to support a possible future pregnancy—needs all the help it can muster. The corpus luteum has a very high metabolic rate, with equally high requirements for blood and oxygen. It pro-duces progesterone, which assists in implantation of the preg-nancy.

It is more than likely that our modern lifestyle has taken us away from what was meant to be a naturally sleepy and lazy time. Newly pregnant women may find they suffer chronic tiredness, whether they are rushing to work or looking after a toddler at home. Whatever you can do to reduce your stress levels at this all-important time in the pregnancy will be of great help. You want to give your baby the best possible chance in the beginning.

Remember, I am talking about patients who miscarry. Please don't misunderstand me: not every woman has to stay in bed the whole time. I'm also not talking about spending 24 hours in your pajamas for the average pregnancy. What I am talking about is lying around, reading a magazine or a book, watching TV, talking on the phone, just reclining. If there are any signs of a threatened miscarriage, *don't go in to work.*

Not only will you feel better for relaxing, but also there is no doubt in my mind that it helps the pregnancy. So if you have previously miscarried or are fearful, then take action yourself when next you become pregnant. *Discuss it with your doctor.* You don't have to give up work altogether; just try to organize a less-pressured schedule. Make sure you sit with your feet up for several hours a day—either while still at work, by taking off early, or by arranging to do some of your work at home.

In fact, I have often wondered why in completely normal, un-complicated pregnancies women, with the consent of their employers and insurance companies, stop working in the last weeks of their pregnancies. It would seem more sensible and more beneficial to take time off in the *early* weeks, when they are feeling tired, irritable, nauseated, and possibly unable to cope with the demands of work.

My last point in favor of bed rest is that it certainly can do no harm, though you must remember to move your legs and change positions to avoid the risk of blood clots. In itself, it is not expensive, though of course giving up work for several weeks or months may prove to be too costly for you and your partner. Or, if you already have a toddler at home and this is a second pregnancy, bed rest may mean hiring someone to help at home. So, yes, there are definitely related expenses. But I know from working with women who have suffered miscarriages that most would do anything to help produce a healthy, full-term baby.

What About Sexual Intercourse?

I'm sure it is hardly necessary to point out that intercourse is inadvisable in early pregnancy if you are experiencing cramping or bleeding or have a history of recurrent miscarriages. Having had intercourse the night before spotting began is *not* likely to be the cause of the threatened miscarriage. But it is known that prostaglandins in semen can stimulate uterine muscle activity and therefore increase contractions. If you have noticed any danger signals, you'd be better off abstaining until your doctor feels the pregnancy is secure. Do discuss it with your doctor, however, if you and your husband desire intercourse, as this may still be the best way to alleviate your anxieties and feel you are communicating well as a couple. My advice would then be to avoid deep penetration and to use condoms so the semen does not enter the vagina.

One other reason for abstaining is that bacteria can be carried on the sperm. If your cervix is short or open (that is, if you have a weak or incompetent cervix), the sperm may enter the uterus through the cervix, possibly infecting the amniotic sac membranes and then the fetus. It is noteworthy that the human female is the only mammal who mates during pregnancy.

How Often Should You See Your Doctor?

I want to emphasize that your relationship with your doctor may be significant to the outcome of your pregnancy if you have previously miscarried. You should be looked after by a doctor whom you like and respect, who is available to you, who will answer your phone calls, and who will treat you without minimizing your concerns.

A woman who has miscarried more than once may need to be seen more often by her physician, even as much as once or twice a week in early pregnancy if need be. The reassurance of knowing your doctor is involved and cares is, in itself, a great stress reducer. Just to be able to voice your fears, or to be seen regularly, will ease your mind.

Reassurance that everything will be all right—because your doctor is accessible—is often the best medicine. For example, someone having an asthma attack may begin to feel better as soon as she is seen by a doctor, even before she is given the medicine to break the attack. We're noticing a similar effect on women who have gone into premature labor. After 28 weeks, if a woman begins early labor contractions, she may find that just reaching the hospital—and being seen by the doctors and nurses—helps the contractions subside, even before being put on medication (which ultimately may not be needed).

What Do the Different Terms Used for a Miscarriage Mean?

Spontaneous Abortion

The terminology relating to miscarriage is surprisingly confusing to most people. For example, the term *spontaneous abortion* is synonymous in medicine with miscarriage. I know it is upsetting to hear the term *abortion* in relation to your much-desired pregnancy, and some women have been heartbroken to read on their records the diagnosis "spontaneous abortion," after the tragic early loss of a pregnancy, but until the medical profession makes a distinction between the two terms, remember that they are interchangeable.

Threatened Miscarriage

If you are suffering from cramping and bleeding, you are more than likely to be told that you have a "threatened abortion" or a "threatened miscarriage."

The term *threatened abortion*, or miscarriage, refers to a situation in early pregnancy in which you have lost some blood and may feel some very slight cramping. It is usually painless, though. The blood is often bright red or may be brown. As I described earlier, this is very common, occurring in 60 to 70 percent of pregnancies, and it usually settles down on its own.

If the pregnancy proceeds, you don't have to worry about the bleeding adversely affecting the baby, since the blood comes from unoccupied areas of the uterus, not from the fetus itself. All studies have shown that bleeding in early pregnancy does not cause any abnormality to the baby; the chances of having a normal healthy baby are the same as if no bleeding had occurred. However, it may cause the baby to weigh slightly less at birth. So unless the bleeding becomes heavy, don't panic. Do go to bed and call your doctor during normal working hours. If, however, the bleeding increases, then you should call your doctor at any time.

Inevitable Miscarriage

If the bleeding becomes heavier and is accompanied by severe cramping, the uterus may already be expelling the fetus. When your doctor examines you, he or she may find that the cervix is already opening, at which point you may be told that the miscarriage is *inevitable*. Although this can sound harsh and cold to you, it is a medical term meaning that there really is little hope of saving the pregnancy. You will probably be offered a D&C, which will require hospitalization and general anesthetic, as the cervix, which is closed, must be dilated before the uterus can be emptied. This would be preferable to going home and enduring cramps until the miscarriage occurs naturally. Even so, you still might require an aspiration if some tissue is left behind. This is an office procedure, as the cervix will not have to be dilated, having already opened for the passing of the pregnancy tissue. If your pregnancy is slightly more advanced, beyond 9 weeks, and you are told that you are going to miscarry, your doctor will probably advise you not to go home, where you would await the natural abortion. Rather, you will be encouraged to have a D&C, either in your doctor's office if he has the necessary facilities or at the hospital to avoid a potential emergency situation from heavy bleeding.

Collecting the Tissue

This is hardly pleasant, but I must emphasize that if you find yourself miscarrying at home, it is advisable to collect the pregnancy tissue when possible. Even though you may not be able to distinguish tissue from blood clots, the best advice is to collect all that is expelled in a clean sterile container, adding only sterile saline (contact lens solution) if available. You can sterilize a clean glass jar and lid by bringing them to a boil in a pan of water and then allowing them to cool. The tissue sample can be stored in the refrigerator, not the freezer, for a few hours if necessary. The sample will help your doctor decide whether you have miscarried or not. Your doctor may also want to send it to pathology for tissue and genetic analysis.

Some miscarriages are caused by genetic, or chromosomal, abnormalities. If this is found to be the cause of your miscarriage, then at least you can be reassured that, first, a cause was found and, second, that it is *unlikely* to recur. Contrary to popular belief, if a chromosomal defect is discovered, particularly in a first pregnancy, it seldom happens again.

Fetal tissue (and other products of conception) can be examined at a pathology laboratory. The information can be of help to you in future pregnancies, as it can offer clues as to why the pregnancy ended, such as clotting, infection, or immune changes. This is an important new area of miscarriage research. In a slightly more advanced pregnancy, a wholly formed fetus can also be checked for normal structural development, such as of the heart and lungs. The placenta, too, may be sent to a pathologist where it will be tested for infections and normal development. New research suggests that blood clots blocking placental vessels may cause early (and late) miscarriages. Miscarriage tissue examination and analysis is providing significant information even from very early pregnancy loss.

Before moving on to describe what doctors mean by the sometimes confusing terms *missed abortion* (or miscarriage) and *blighted ovum,* I would like you to read about Ruth, who has undergone a variety of miscarriages, and other problems with infertility—a mixture that can occur particularly with mothers who delay childbearing. She was able during one miscarriage to save the fetal tissue. I think her straightforward way of describing this experience will be helpful.

Ruth has had five miscarriages, but now she has three healthy young children. She and her husband seem determined to have a large family, for she is now pregnant with her fourth. But without proper care and treatment by her doctors, her story could have been very different.

"I Began to Go a Little Crazy . . ."

Around ten years ago, when I was 29, I had my first miscarriage. It seemed quite a normal thing to happen, fairly early in the first trimester, at about 8 to 10 weeks of pregnancy. It wasn't very traumatic because I felt it could happen to anyone. And it was not very long before I was pregnant again. But I lost that one, too. They were both the same, happening at about 10 weeks.

My doctor had said he could do nothing until I'd lost three. So I became pregnant again, and this third one was very traumatic. It happened at 8 weeks, and the important part was that it was the *third* time. I'd begun bleeding over the weekend, and when I went in to see the doctor he examined me and said the tissue was in my vagina, and he removed the tissue with forceps. When I walked out of his office, I was in such an emotional state, I never thought to ask if the tissue could be tested. So it was never sent for genetics analysis to find a cause.

I found another doctor whom I consulted three weeks after the miscarriage because I wasn't feeling well. He informed me that I was still pregnant. In fact, I'd been pregnant with twins and there was still one sac inside. He tried to help me, but again I started bleeding at home and eventually miscarried at 12 weeks. There was a lot of blood and the cramping was pretty bad. I lay down most of the time, but in the end I went and sat on the toilet. I knew I had to be careful and collect the fetus. I recognized when it was passing because it felt slippery as it was coming out. The fetus seemed to be in a little bag, separate from the blood. I collected it and put it in a plastic container. But, as you can imagine, I was very upset by the whole experience. Now that I'd actually seen the baby, it was no longer just blood that I was losing, but a child.

At that point I began to go a little crazy. I appeared calm on the surface, but inside I was desperately trying to keep control of my emotions. I took my container in to the doctor, feeling very weak. He sent it for testing, but the results didn't give any clue as to why I had miscarried. I then became pregnant again, and this time the doctor gave me shots of HCG [human chorionic gonadotropin] from the start of the pregnancy. At 16 weeks, I went for an amniocentesis appointment. On the ultrasound examination, which takes place before the amniocentesis, they saw that the baby had been dead for about a week. My pregnancy symptoms had started to go away, so I suppose I'd been suspicious. But I could not understand why it had suddenly died, because this time I had even gone beyond the first 3 months. It was awful having to face up to it before the sonographer. The doctor seemed vague and his explanation did not help. I sensed he felt bad and didn't know how to deal with the situation. I was given a D&C to empty my uterus. The pathology report on the tissue did not tell why I had lost the pregnancy.

All these miscarriages were with my first husband, and a geneticist found nothing wrong with either of us. So there were still no explanations. I was told to keep on trying. But I didn't want to try anymore. Psychologically, at that point, I couldn't do it again.

But life went on, and I don't know if it had anything to do

with all those miscarriages, but my marriage broke up. Then, five years ago, I remarried. Within three months I was pregnant. We both desperately wanted children, and I was referred to a doctor who was particularly interested in miscarriages. I was already on progesterone from my former doctor, though my progesterone levels on the blood tests were not low. But I was left on progesterone as a precaution. This time, I went through to 26 weeks, when premature labor started. I was rushed to the hospital, given an intravenous infusion, and put on ritodrine, a drug used to relax the uterus and control the contractions. It worked well, and, once the contractions settled down, I was discharged home, where I was kept on oral ritodrine tablets.

At 33 weeks, I went into labor spontaneously. My daughter was born healthy and fine at 4 pounds 2 ounces. Now, at least, I knew I could have a baby. I really wanted to keep on trying for a larger family. So, five months later, I became pregnant again. We just decided we'd better get a move on, as I was then 34. My husband has a good career, and luckily I don't need to work. My son went to 36 weeks, and he was born healthy and fine. Both of my babies, however, have had to stay in the neonatal care unit for about three weeks because of slight breathing problems.

My third baby, for whose pregnancy I was also given progesterone and ritodrine, was born at 33 weeks. We still wanted more children, and I became pregnant again. But this time, at 6 weeks, I suddenly didn't feel pregnant again. On the sonogram, we saw an empty pregnancy sac, a blighted ovum. I wasn't really very upset, as I had my three children. But then I had a second blighted ovum, in the next pregnancy, which is unusual because I was told it doesn't tend to happen a second time.

So by then I was 38 and worried I couldn't get pregnant anymore, as I had been trying for three years. I had to turn to an infertility specialist and was put on a low dosage of a fertility tablet called Clomid. Before we were married, my husband had been tested, and his sperm motility was found to be very low. He was put on steroids and a high dosage of vitamin C. And as that had seemed to work before, the doctor suggested that we try the same method again. It was successful, and now I'm 6 months pregnant again. I've been on ritodrine since 21 weeks and was on progesterone vaginal suppositories for the first 3 months. Again my uterus is contracting early.

Every time I go into a pregnancy, it's nerve-wracking for the first 3 months, because we still don't know for certain what has caused the miscarriages. The anxiety—and confusion over what is really happening—eats away at you. I hope my attempt at giving a medical account of my pregnancies hasn't been too confusing!

☘

Missed Abortion

Ruth's experience, which fortunately ended happily, included two other types of miscarriages known in medical terms as a *missed abortion* and a *blighted ovum*. A missed abortion—you will seldom hear it referred to as a missed miscarriage, maybe simply because of the clumsy alliteration—refers to a fetus that has died but has not been expelled (see Figure 1). The fetal and placental tissue are still inside you. If this happens, it is advisable to have a D&C, either at your doctor's office or at the hospital, without too

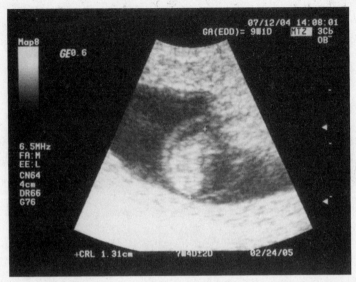

Figure 1. This is an ultrasound photograph of a missed abortion. The embryo shown did not have a heartbeat. A normal embryo would also show more body contours.

much delay. The fetal material can be taken straight to the hospital or directed to the correct lab for chromosomal testing and pathology. Some tissue can also be sent to a placental pathologist to look for the immediate cause of the embryo's death: for example, clotting and infection. This critical analysis is useful in treating and managing of future pregnancies. The fresher the tissue, the more likely we are to receive usable results; it can be difficult for the laboratory to grow the chromosomes if the tissue has been dead too long.

And if tissue is collected as soon as possible, you will not have to suffer the potentially traumatic experience of going home, knowing you have a dead baby inside of you. You will avoid a remote risk of infection getting into the uterus and harming you. You will also avoid the risk of the fetus aborting itself during the night, with the consequent emergency rush to the hospital. Lastly, there is the very remote risk of your developing a clotting disorder if a dead fetus is retained beyond about 6 weeks. This is especially so with a more advanced fetal death, rather than in a very early pregnancy.

Obtaining the tissue for examination is very important, despite the fear expressed by many patients of adhesions or scars forming in the womb that would interfere with future pregnancies. If you have suffered recurrent miscarriages, it is vital for you and your husband to find out the possible cause. The information will also help your doctor determine your future treatment next time you become pregnant.

If you have had a previous D&C, the tissue can be removed very gently by a technique similar to CVS, under ultrasound guidance, to decrease the chance of adhesions forming. There is also a very new procedure, embryoscopy, whereby a narrow viewing tube called a hysteroscope is inserted through the cervix to inspect the pregnancy sac. This may allow the doctor to see if there are structural abnormalities of the embryo (the advantage is lost once removal is undertaken). Embryoscopy can also aid with the gentle removal of the pregnancy sac, minimizing adhesions.

What Is a Blighted Ovum?

A blighted ovum means there is no fetus inside the pregnancy sac (see Figure 2).

Normally, a fertilized egg develops in two different directions: one mass of cells forms the pregnancy sac and the other forms the embryo. In the case of a blighted ovum, the second stage just does not happen: pregnancy hormone levels rise, the pregnancy sac develops, but the embryo does not. You can liken it to grow-

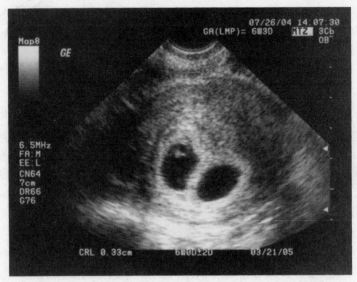

Figure 2. This ultrasound photograph taken at six weeks of
pregnancy with twins shows a blighted ovum. The pregnancy
sac on the left shows a normal pregnancy. The pregnancy sac on
the right is empty, filled only with fluid (dark area in center).

ing beans and waiting for the sprouts to shoot through. Some just
do not take. Roots may develop but there are no stems.

Weeks may go by without bleeding or signs of miscarriage.
After a while you may have a very dark brown discharge, and your
breasts may stop feeling as swollen or sensitive as before. You
probably won't miscarry spontaneously for a long time. The
blighted ovum may not be discovered until you visit your doctor
and have an ultrasound scan to look for the fetal heartbeat.

Blighted ova, which are thought to be caused by a lack of
chromosomes in either a sperm or an egg, are more common in
older couples. One of the reasons why we are seeing more
blighted ova these days is that we use ultrasound more often in
early pregnancy and can therefore detect the empty sac. Also, as

parents today tend to delay childbearing, there is an increased risk of a miscarriage from poor egg or sperm quality.

In the past, doctors were often unable to explain why a pregnancy was not developing. Now, fortunately, we can tell what has happened by using sonography, but we still can do nothing to save a blighted ovum. With no embryo present, there is obviously nothing that can be done.

With ultrasound, we are becoming more aware of certain eventualities. For example, your doctor may see three or four empty sacs inside the uterus. Some women may be conceiving multiple blighted ova. Women have hundreds of thousands of eggs, and men have millions of sperm, and it seems that, more often than we realized, more than one egg is fertilized at the same time.

We are aware now of a phenomenon called the "vanishing twin." A twin pregnancy is diagnosed; then, after some vaginal bleeding, a repeat sonogram shows that one of the twins has disappeared (or miscarried) while the other continues to grow normally.

As mentioned earlier, ultrasound has become more sophisticated. The transvaginal probe has been developed, which, when inserted into the vagina right up against the uterus, can detect very early pregnancies in some detail. This means we can diagnose a normal continuing pregnancy much earlier than was previously possible, and thus eliminate the diagnosis of a blighted ovum early on.

Preparing Yourself Mentally to Cope with a Missed Abortion or Blighted Ovum

If the information from an ultrasound scan confirms that the pregnancy will not continue—either because the fetus is already dead (missed abortion) or because there is an empty sac in the uterus (blighted ovum)—the doctor may initially seem concerned mainly about your health and physical condition and will probably spend less time (of necessity) on your sadness and grieving. This is not an easy time emotionally, even under the best conditions, but you must realize that medical management of your situation has to be the first priority. It pays to listen to and have confidence in your doctor.

In all likelihood, your doctor will recommend performing a D&C in his or her office, or in the hospital, and will explain how the uterus has to be emptied. The other method of management would be to let the fetus expel itself from your uterus spontaneously. However, it is emotionally difficult for a woman to carry a dead fetus. Further, bear in mind that holding on to a nonviable pregnancy will only delay the return of your menstrual cycle and the next opportunity for you to attempt another pregnancy. Also, if the miscarriage occurs spontaneously, it is possible that pregnancy tissue may be trapped in the mouth of the womb, or cervix. This would lead to heavy bleeding and emergency surgery, which should be avoided if at all possible.

Other Reasons for Bleeding in Early Pregnancy

Molar Pregnancy (hydatidiform mole)
Molar pregnancy is a rare condition that starts off like a normal pregnancy; but then, at about 10 weeks or so, irregular vaginal bleeding occurs, which may be heavy and even cause anemia. Profuse vomiting and severe nausea are also common symptoms. When the doctor examines you, the uterus, as well as the ovaries, may seem overly large. High blood pressure (pre-eclampsia) may also develop.

Another indication of molar pregnancy is high levels of the pregnancy hormone HCG (human chorionic gonadotropin). The condition may be caused by chromosomal abnormalities of the egg or sperm. The placental tissue grows inordinately fast, producing a mass of cysts, like a bunch of grapes. The rapid growth of the placenta raises hormone levels beyond what is normal, which is what leads to excessive vomiting and high blood pressure. It is a benign condition that is more common in patients in their early teens or those nearing 40. Occasionally, the little cysts resembling grapes may be passed vaginally.

Bleeding may be the first sign, but it may not start until quite late, even beyond the 16th week of pregnancy. The blood is usually very dark and has been described as prune-colored. The condition may be discovered by sonogram at an earlier stage. Fortunately, this condition is rare, occurring in only 1 out of 1200 pregnancies in the United States and Europe.

Although the mole would eventually miscarry spontaneously, a D&C is recommended to ensure that all the tissue from the pregnancy is removed from the uterus. There is a small chance that this condition can become cancerous. *Choriocarcinoma*, as it is then called, affects only about 10 percent of molar pregnancies and is completely curable.

Because of the risks involved—the tissue may start growing elsewhere in the body or, rarely, may become malignant—your doctor will continue to follow your condition, mainly through blood tests, for up to a year after the D&C. Women are usually advised to wait a year before trying to conceive again. The birth control pill is the preferred form of contraception. If the blood test results continue to prove normal after a year, you may resume plans to conceive.

A diagnosis of molar pregnancy can be very scary. Not only do you have to undergo a strange, and hardly talked about, form of miscarriage, but it carries with it the remote risk of cancer.

There is also the slight risk of a molar pregnancy recurring, so the next time around your doctor will monitor your pregnancy very carefully in the early weeks. But it is important to remember that this is a rare condition.

Ectopic or Tubal Pregnancy

Although an ectopic pregnancy is not a miscarriage, it is regarded as such because the pregnancy does not continue and often the early symptoms are similar. You should be aware of the difference, however, as an ectopic pregnancy can seriously damage the fallopian tube, may affect your future fertility, and could ultimately rupture the tube, endangering your life through acute blood loss.

No one is quite sure why ectopic pregnancies happen, but the fertilized ovum may have taken too long to travel down the fallopian tube and, on the 7th day, instead of reaching the uterus where it should implant, it embeds itself in the tube where the beginnings of a pregnancy are acted out.

Pregnancy hormones are produced at sufficient levels to make you miss a period and produce a positive pregnancy test. The condition may not be discovered until your first visit to the doctor. An internal examination will reveal that the uterus has not expanded as in a normal pregnancy. An ultrasound scan will not always show the pregnancy in the tube, but it will show the uterus to be empty.

Symptoms to watch out for are the lack of pregnancy symptoms or less nausea or vomiting than in normal pregnancy; some cramping in the lower abdomen; and slight spotting or staining of blood. Other indicators are a feeling of dizziness and shoulder-tip pain. If such pain or bleeding persists, you must report to your doctor or the hospital, as you don't want to delay the diagnosis. But remember, too, that tubal pregnancy is fairly rare, and the diagnosis will probably be of a normal pregnancy, and your worries will have been for nothing.

With early diagnosis, an ectopic pregnancy can be treated medically with drugs (methotrexate), avoiding the necessity for surgery. But if the ectopic is too far advanced for drug treatment, then surgery will be necessary. So, if you have noticed a missed period, associated with low cramplike abdominal pain and scant or dark spotting, do see your doctor as quickly as possible, particularly if you have a history of high-risk factors, such as the past or present use of an intrauterine device or infection in your tubes (salpingitis), which may promote tubal pregnancies.

Your doctor will diagnose a tubal pregnancy by monitoring hormone levels in your blood (they normally double every 48 hours) and also by using abdominal or transvaginal sonography. If surgery is necessary, and depending on your particular medical situation, your doctor will either use laparoscopy, which does not require opening the abdomen, or laparotomy, which requires a wide incision to open the abdomen. Both of these surgical procedures require hospitalization and are done in an operating room under general anesthesia. Unless it is a dire emergency, you will be admitted on the morning of the procedure, not having eaten or drunk from midnight of that day.

Laparoscopy is the least invasive procedure. In the operating room, the gynecologist distends your abdomen with carbon dioxide gas, through a needle inserted below your belly button, and then passes a viewing instrument (laparoscope) through a tiny incision in your umbilicus. Additional probes are placed through small puncture wounds (at the pubic hair line) to help the doctor to move your organs for better inspection and to assist in removing the pregnancy from the fallopian tube. The operation takes about 45 minutes to one hour. You can usually leave the hospital after a few hours in the recovery room. Occasionally you may have to remain in the hospital overnight. The stitches do not usually require removal.

Complete Abortion

If your doctor informs you that there has been a "complete abortion," this means the miscarriage has brought out all fetal tissue and the uterus is empty. There will be no need for a D&C. If you are bleeding, you may be given ergometrine tablets by mouth to help the uterus contract and so reduce the amount of blood loss.

"Emptying" the Uterus

If the miscarriage has not completely expelled the fetal tissue, how the uterus is "emptied" depends on the stage of the pregnancy. If your miscarriage occurred under 8 weeks or if the cervix is dilated from the passage of fetal tissue, a suction curettage can be performed in your doctor's office using a local anesthetic in the cervix. Some Demerol (or Pethidine) may be given intravenously as a painkiller.

In a hospital D&C procedure, the uterus may be suctioned or curetted, and a general anesthetic may be required if your pregnancy was advanced. Otherwise, only intravenous sedation may be used. Antibiotics are not usually given unless you have a fever or there is suspicion of an infection.

Sometimes the tissue is sent by your doctor to the genetics lab for chromosome analysis, especially if you have previously miscarried. The D&C will also give your doctor the chance to investigate the inside of your uterus for any structural abnormalities. A follow-up visit is usually arranged for two weeks after the procedure so that your doctor can make sure your uterus has returned to normal size and there is no infection. Then you can discuss future plans.

If you miscarried beyond about 12 weeks and the fetal tissue is retained, the cervix can be softened, or "ripened," usually overnight, with a prostaglandin gel or tablet placed at the top of the vagina. This avoids the need for a forcible dilatation. After this procedure a slight further dilatation will usually be necessary, and the uterus can be curetted or suctioned to empty it, without the risk of damage to the cervix.

Laminaria (dried seaweed sticks) may also be inserted into the cervix by the doctor the night before you go into the hospital. Insertion takes only a few minutes and may cause mild cramps, which sometimes continue through the night. The dried seaweed swells and thus gradually opens the cervix, facilitating the D&C the next day. These are great advances in technique, allowing fewer complications.

Suppositories containing prostaglandins may also be inserted into the vagina every four hours. This induces a minilabor and an eventual miscarriage, with expulsion of the pregnancy from the uterus. This must be done in a hospital and may take many hours. Prostaglandins may cause marked gastrointestinal side effects such as nausea or vomiting. The procedure may also need to be followed by a D&C, as tissue is often retained when this method is used. It is, therefore, less popular than the previous two methods described.

After your uterus has been emptied, bleeding may last for a few days or up to two weeks. However, it should not be very heavy. To avoid infection, use pads, not tampons, and do not have sexual intercourse for two weeks. Any fever over 100 degrees Fahrenheit should be reported to your doctor. Your period should return within four to six weeks after the D&C, but it may take longer depending on how far your pregnancy had progressed.

What Is the Association Between
Miscarriage and Parental Age?

The older a woman is, the greater the likelihood of miscarriage. This does not seem to prevent women today from attempting a pregnancy in their late thirties or forties. But there is no way around the facts. Men, and especially women, in their late thirties and older:

- are more at risk for developing degenerative diseases such as high blood pressure or diabetes
- usually have more responsibility and potentially higher stress levels from their careers
- are at greater risk of chromosomal abnormalities in their offspring—hence the recommendation to have the baby's chromosomes tested by amniocentesis, or chorionic villus sampling (if the mother is over 35)

As you will read in Margaret's and Phoebe's stories, however, there is plenty of true grit and determination in such women.

"Whether There Ever Was a Fetus or Not,
the Buildup Is the Same"

Margaret is a lively woman who runs her own business. She had suffered through three miscarriages, all of which were blighted ova. At one time she was afraid she might never have a baby because she and her husband are both over 40.

I wasn't married until I was 38. Neither my husband nor I had been married before, which must make us most unusual. To make matters even stranger, I'd never been pregnant. Raised a strict Catholic, I was a virgin until I was 30 years old, which must make me sound archaic!

But now here I was happily married, and we wanted to try to get pregnant almost immediately. But it took three years before I conceived. Maybe we just weren't having sex often enough, since we were a two-career couple getting on somewhat in years. However, ultimately I did get pregnant and we were both thrilled.

The pregnancy began in May, and I miscarried at 12 weeks, on my mother's birthday. I'll never forget the day, because I'd just told her the good news. I began spotting over the weekend. I was in touch with my doctor, who advised me to go to bed. I lost the baby during the weekend. I tried to collect what was coming out, but that felt like a bizarre thing to be doing. I couldn't imagine what I was going to get. There I was in the bathroom, holding a cup. I did collect some clots.

I'd been warned I was at some risk during pregnancy, as I was over 40 years old. But we had not expected this to happen. I went into the doctor's office, and I remember sitting there thinking about everything. It all seemed so strange, like a bad dream. The sonogram showed it was a blighted ovum, just an empty sac. Since my blood is Rh-negative, he performed a D&C, followed by a shot of anti-D [an injection designed to destroy Rh-positive cells, which may cause sensitization and antibodies that may attack the next pregnancy].

I think my husband was angry, or at least he was trying not to be angry with me, that maybe I hadn't taken enough care of myself. Whether there was ever a fetus or not, the psychological buildup is just the same. I was so sad and had to go through a lot of mourning before I felt ready to try again.

The second miscarriage was the hardest because there was such a sense of loss. I was in my forties and pregnant again. This really felt like our last chance, and we both wanted a child so badly. Losing the pregnancy was losing the dream of the child in our lives. I can verify that it takes about 30 seconds, from the moment you're given the positive result of a pregnancy test to dressing the baby in clothes and going out to the park, in your mind. Anyway, this one was also a blighted ovum, which I lost in the 10th to the 11th week. Then, within a short space of time, I had a third miscarriage, another blighted ovum, discovered in the 6th to 8th week.

There really is no way of logically convincing yourself it was not a child you lost, because in those weeks of imaginings, as far as you knew, the child inside of you had so many possibilities. The pain still comes from the lost dream. To you, it's a baby that has died.

Miraculously, our next pregnancy—after waiting three months—seemed good. There was some slight spotting again, over which I panicked, of course, and took myself to bed. Since the progesterone level in my blood was low, I was put on vaginal suppositories and advised to rest as much as possible. I brought all my work back home for the first three months. It was Christmas and I really wanted to go out for dinner. I phoned the doctor to ask if it would be all right. He said very firmly, "No. You stay home." At my age, he felt it was sensible to be as careful as is humanly possible.

Apart from some gas pains and a little cramping, all went well. When I was 6 months pregnant, everything was so good we even went on vacation. At the end, I went 11 days past my due date when my water broke. I was induced and our son was born, normal and healthy. He's like a gift from God to us.

ϒ

"I Could Sense That My Body Was Attacking the Embryos"

For Phoebe, it has also been a long journey. Now 41, she and her husband started trying to get pregnant five years ago. They have just brought home their 1-week-old baby, born at 33½ weeks, weighing 5 pounds 12 ounces and measuring 17 inches long. Phoebe is a sophisticated communications specialist at a research agency who lives in Washington, D.C. When she heard about a doctor in New York City who could help her, she had no qualms about making the time for that appointment.

ϒ

I knew I was losing babies, I could even sense that my body was attacking the embryos. Every time we went through the IVF process, the eggs were good, but implantation failed. It's so painful to think that we went through all that for years. Then, when I went to see the new doctor, within 10 minutes he said, "You have an autoimmune problem and without treatment you'll never keep a pregnancy." He came up with a treatment plan. Three weeks later I was pregnant, and we now have a healthy, lively baby girl!

I'd been lulled into that "you can do it later in life—you can have it all" Hollywood mentality. It never occurred to me I'd have turned 40 years before having my first baby. I started trying to conceive when I was 36. At first, when nothing happened, my regular ob/gyn just said to keep trying, it would be okay. I was finally referred to an endocrinologist, who claimed it must be my eggs, because I was already getting quite old. We asked whether it might be related to immunologic disorders, because I had been through chronic fatigue syndrome. But he shook his head.

We started on IVF. After the third cycle, I became pregnant. But I lost the baby right away, at 5 weeks. I could "feel" my body attacking the pregnancy. By that time I had joined an online support group called www.IVFconnections.com. Women join up from all over the world. Many have been trying for a long time. Thanks to the perseverance of these smart, determined women, and physicians like Dr. Scher, many of us "hopeless cases" now have babies.

We did two more cycles and I remember getting positive pregnancy results on a home testing kit, but then it would be lost. It was such a painful process to be losing babies like this. My embryos looked good. They were graded on average a 2 (with a 1 being the best quality and a 4 being poor quality). On the surface there was no real reason for me not to get pregnant. The IVF doctor ran a lot of tests but would not do serious immunologic testing. By May last year, based on my research online and talking to other women, we told our doctor that we really wanted to go for full immunologic testing. I gave them a long list of tests that I felt should be done, including the endometrial function test. My doctor in Washington agreed to do the tests, but when the results came back showing abnormal results in a host of categories, his advice was to pursue donor eggs and ignore the test results.

I knew of no one in this city who could analyze the test results and help us come up with a plan. We contacted the doctor in New York and in August my husband and I were given an appointment. Within 10 minutes, he said, "You may have an autoimmune problem and without treatment you'll probably never keep a pregnancy." He suggested a diagnosis and ran additional tests. As I guessed, my body was attacking the embryo each time at the moment of implantation, because I had high levels of natural killer cells, which can do this, and mild endometriosis, also an immune condition. I also had a blood-clotting factor and was prescribed Lovenox (heparin) for this; I was put on baby aspirin and folic acid too. I also had IVIG treatments, which help to correct immune problems. Three weeks later I became pregnant. Fortunately, I only needed IVIG up to 16 weeks, as by then the NK cells were back to normal. I was able to stop the Lovenox at 25 weeks.

I continued my prenatal care in Washington, but I would often phone the New York office for advice. They were so kind and understanding and just let me talk or ask questions. I only went back there one more time. The baby came 6½ weeks early, as I had placenta previa and had to have an emergency C-section.

I really want to help other women now. I feel I wasted four precious years and, without the complete testing, I wouldn't have a baby now. Once you turn 40, it certainly drives home the urgency of age and getting pregnant. I know so many doctors are against the idea of immunologic testing and treatment, but I just can't understand why in such difficult cases. I also can't understand why insurance companies are prepared to fund three to six repeatedly failing cycles of IVF, which might be a complete waste of money, without the immunologic tests and treatment. We call our baby the $100,000 miracle! While she'll always be a miracle to us, the cost could have been a fraction of that, financially and emotionally.

❦

What Causes Midtrimester Miscarriages?

The majority of miscarriages happen before the 12th to 14th week of pregnancy, but as we have seen in the stories shared so far, many women also undergo stressful late miscarriages and even lose a baby they have already felt kicking. These movements are usually felt from 18 to 20 weeks of pregnancy and onward.

Late miscarriages are usually not due to hormonal insufficiency because, from about the 10th to 11th week of pregnancy, the placenta begins to support the fetus with adequate levels of progesterone and other hormones. An incompetent or weak cervix is an important cause of miscarriages after the 12th to 16th week. The cervix opens and the membranes rupture, either because infection reaches the membranes from the vagina, or because of undue pressure on the cervix, possibly from an abnormally shaped uterus.

Another cause of a late miscarriage may be a multiple pregnancy: two, three, or more fetuses may overdistend the uterus to such an extent that the cervix begins to open, though this would not usually happen until after the 20th week. A second-trimester loss can also be caused by interference in the blood flow to the fetus from antibodies in the blood, for example anticardiolipin antibodies, which cause clotting.

Unlike first-trimester miscarriages, which begin with cramping and bleeding, middle-trimester losses due to an incompetent cervix usually begin with the passage of amniotic fluid from ruptured membranes or a painless gush of fresh blood. On examination, the cervix is often found to be dilated. The miscarriage then usually proceeds quickly and somewhat painlessly over a very short period of time—hours rather than days—in contrast to the earlier, prolonged, and painful miscarriages under 12 weeks.

Providing the membranes have not ruptured and the cervix is

less than 3 centimeters dilated when the patient is examined, it may be possible even at this late stage for your doctor to close off the cervix by placing a stitch in it, thus enabling the pregnancy to continue. But if there are contractions or bleeding, your doctor will not even attempt to put in the stitch until these have settled down.

Sometimes in the midtrimester the fetus may die, but be retained. Or it may be expelled following a period of bleeding and cramping. This type of late-pregnancy loss may be due to the presence of antibodies that are inherited (thrombophilias) or acquired (such as anticardiolipin antibodies). The antibodies cause blood clotting, which interferes with the baby's blood supply across the placenta. They can be diagnosed and treated with heparin, a blood-thinning drug, and baby aspirin.

The Role of Beta-Mimetic Drugs in Middle-Trimester Threatened Miscarriage

Beta-mimetic drugs (for example, Terbutaline) have been approved for use by women who are more than 20 weeks pregnant to stop contractions of the uterus. Their main use is in treating premature labor, when contractions begin before the baby is mature enough to live outside the womb.

Beta-mimetics are safe for the baby. The only side effect on the mother is that they cause her heart to beat very fast. They will not cause damage to the heart, just the discomfort of a racing feeling. When fully advised of the side effect, most women find it tolerable. It tends to disappear if the patient remains on the medication for a long time.

When a stitch is placed in the cervix to treat an incompetent cervix, and undue contractions are noticed, bed rest will be advised, and indomethacin tablets or rectal suppositories (or Terbu-

taline if the pregnancy is over 20 weeks) may be prescribed to set-
tle the contractions down.

While drinking is not recommended in pregnancy because of
the risk of fetal alcohol syndrome and possible birth defects, an
occasional glass of wine will not harm the fetus and may prove
beneficial in helping relax the uterus in a pregnancy before 20
weeks. But take alcohol only on your doctor's advice.

Stillbirth, or Death in Utero

Any very late death of a fetus, either in the uterus, at birth, or
shortly thereafter, must be one of the hardest experiences for a
parent to deal with. There is no escaping the fact that the closer
the baby comes to delivery, and to survival outside the uterus, the
more violent and cruel will be the shock.

Today, the causes of stillbirth can largely be avoided through
good prenatal care and early induction of labor if the fetus seems
to be in trouble. Indeed, there are times when a baby is safer in
an incubator than in the uterus. The baby may not be receiving
adequate nutrition if, for example, the mother has high blood
pressure.

Severe bleeding late in the pregnancy can also endanger the
baby. Disorders of the placenta that lead to bleeding in late pregnancy are *placenta previa* (where the placenta lies low in the uterus
between the cervix and the fetus's head) and *abruption* (separation
of the placenta from the uterine wall). An abruption can be very
dangerous, potentially leading to the baby's death within a matter
of hours. Therefore, *any* blood loss after the 28th week must be
reported immediately to your doctor and should be investigated.

No one can yet predict an abruption, but we can now attempt
to diagnose it with ultrasound, though this is difficult. Further

treatment will then be arranged, or, if necessary, an immediate delivery will be performed by cesarean section. A placenta previa is not as dramatic and usually presents as repeated small hemorrhages of painless bright red bleeding, from about the 30th to the 32nd week of pregnancy. With a placenta previa the baby is usually delivered by cesarean section as soon as it is mature. An abruption occurs later in pregnancy than a placenta previa, around the 35th week, producing pain and dark bleeding, and the patient may suffer from high blood pressure.

There are rare cases in which the baby becomes entangled in the umbilical cord: it can twist and tighten two or three times around the baby's neck, with fatal results. Or, if the baby has a long cord, it may swim around and through the cord, causing it to knot, which can also be fatal. These cord accidents are, fortunately, very rare.

With good prenatal care you and your doctor can reduce these tragedies, which is why pregnant women should have early and regular prenatal visits. Nevertheless, despite our conscientious approach, stillbirths do happen for which there are simply no obvious explanations.

Ultrasound may help more and more in predicting such tragedies. It is very valuable in detecting growth retardation—for example, from poor nutrition in the uterus (perhaps caused by the mother's raised blood pressure or repeated vaginal bleeding)—by evaluating the baby's weight and size. With ultrasound, we can now diagnose the cause of bleeding in late pregnancy, and we can differentiate placenta previa from abruption, which requires different management. We can also tell if there is a severe fetal abnormality, which may lead to the baby dying in the uterus; in some cases, treatment can even be given to correct and avoid this happening. Fetal abnormalities may be accompanied by abnormal amounts of amniotic fluid—either too much (polyhydramnios) or too little (oligohydramnios); this can be seen on ultrasound. Also in late pregnancy ultrasound can be used to count the number of blood vessels in the baby's umbilical cord (normally three), alerting us to the possibility of fetal abnormalities.

How You Can Keep an Eye on Your Baby's Well-being in Advanced Pregnancy

Now I would like to describe some tests that will give both you and your doctor an accurate idea of just how your baby is doing late in the pregnancy.

Fetal Movement Chart

The first of these is a fetal movement (see Figure 3). The mother uses the chart to record the frequency of the baby's movements. It may give you a much better sense of something abnormal beginning to appear and will increase your knowledge of when to notify the doctor of significant changes.

In early pregnancy, the average number of movements per day is low. But fetal movements can be felt from around the 18th week, this is known as *quickening*. Movements will increase and peak between the 29th and 38th week. The baby's movements in the third trimester are its best expression of well-being. When it is kicking, writhing, and squirming about, then the baby is healthy and happy. In the last two weeks of pregnancy, the style of movements may change from kicking to writhing, as the baby is becoming large in relation to the amount of amniotic fluid it floats in, thus giving it less room to move.

The average number of daily movements made by the fetus and reported by mothers varies from 4 to 1400—quite a difference! Most will vary from 32 to 100 movements per day. There is no significance in the actual number you report, only in the changes to the number (that is, if they suddenly decrease dramatically). In fact, on an ultrasound scan, we can see that the baby is making even more movements than the mother feels. Presumably only those movements that hit the uterine wall are sensed by the mother.

Here's how to keep the chart: Select three convenient times during the day when you can chart the number of movements your baby makes for 30 minutes. Mark down anything you feel—writhing, kicking, or any movement. You might choose, for example, 8:30 to 9:00 A.M., 5:30 to 6:00 P.M., and 10:00 to 10:30 P.M. Choose regular times when you know you can relax and feel the baby—the time after breakfast, lunch, and dinner may also be convenient. The process in itself will be reassuring for you, since by concentrating on the baby's movements you will know everything is going well. These records will also help your doctor assess whether the activity level is adequate for the baby's size and age.

You might learn from the chart that your baby has sleep-wake periods and moves around more in the evening than in the day, and that for certain periods, there are no movements at all. We assume these periods are when the baby is sleeping. The rest periods will not be consistent. Babies in the uterus are not on a regular nap schedule!

There will be no association between the number of movements and your age or the number of previous children you have had. But if you smoke, they may decrease. Various stimuli such as sweet foods or drinks, including orange juice; noise; external light; touch and ultrasound may initiate more fetal movements.

From the 7th month of pregnancy, be ready to report to your doctor or to the hospital any change in fetal movements. You must definitely treat the situation as an emergency if there are only three or four movements, or none at all, over a 12-hour period. Some doctors suggest testing over two hours and find that

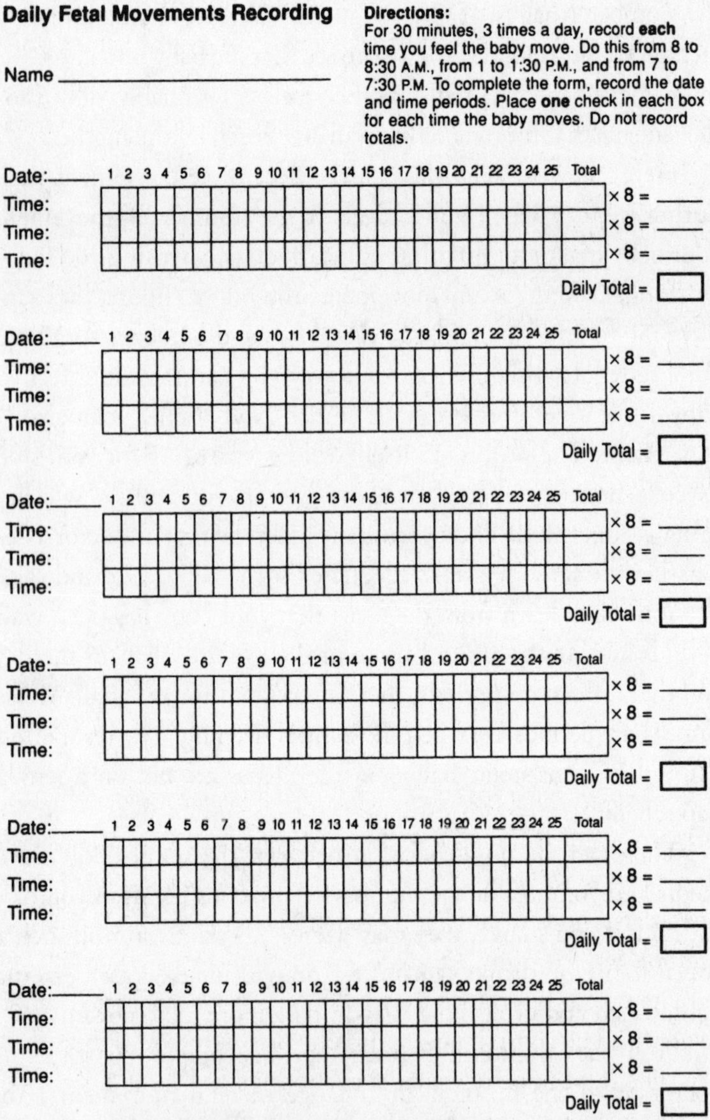

Daily Fetal Movements Recording

Name _____

Directions:
For 30 minutes, 3 times a day, record **each** time you feel the baby move. Do this from 8 to 8:30 A.M., from 1 to 1:30 P.M., and from 7 to 7:30 P.M. To complete the form, record the date and time periods. Place **one** check in each box for each time the baby moves. Do not record totals.

Date:____ 1 2 3 4 5 6 7 8 9 10 11 12 13 14 15 16 17 18 19 20 21 22 23 24 25 Total
Time: × 8 = ____
Time: × 8 = ____
Time: × 8 = ____
                                                                       Daily Total = [   ]

Date:____ 1 2 3 4 5 6 7 8 9 10 11 12 13 14 15 16 17 18 19 20 21 22 23 24 25 Total
Time: × 8 = ____
Time: × 8 = ____
Time: × 8 = ____
                                                                       Daily Total = [   ]

Date:____ 1 2 3 4 5 6 7 8 9 10 11 12 13 14 15 16 17 18 19 20 21 22 23 24 25 Total
Time: × 8 = ____
Time: × 8 = ____
Time: × 8 = ____
                                                                       Daily Total = [   ]

Date:____ 1 2 3 4 5 6 7 8 9 10 11 12 13 14 15 16 17 18 19 20 21 22 23 24 25 Total
Time: × 8 = ____
Time: × 8 = ____
Time: × 8 = ____
                                                                       Daily Total = [   ]

Date:____ 1 2 3 4 5 6 7 8 9 10 11 12 13 14 15 16 17 18 19 20 21 22 23 24 25 Total
Time: × 8 = ____
Time: × 8 = ____
Time: × 8 = ____
                                                                       Daily Total = [   ]

Date:____ 1 2 3 4 5 6 7 8 9 10 11 12 13 14 15 16 17 18 19 20 21 22 23 24 25 Total
Time: × 8 = ____
Time: × 8 = ____
Time: × 8 = ____
                                                                       Daily Total = [   ]

An actual fetal movement chart that you may use, following the instructions at the top of the chart, in collaboration with your doctor.

Figure 3. Fetal movement chart.

10 or more movements during this time is reassuring. Your doctor will be able to follow up your suspicions by nonstress testing or an ultrasound scan. If there have been no movements for some hours, it might mean a problem, but, fortunately, it usually does not. Nevertheless, such a chart is a cheap and easy test that may alert your doctor to a potential problem.

Fetal Stress Test

If your baby's well-being is in question in the third trimester of pregnancy, there are two types of stress tests that can be performed for reassurance. *Nonstress testing* (NST) will show that when the baby moves, its heart rate also increases. Before a nonstress test, you should not smoke, take any sedating drugs, or drink alcohol. Have something to eat, preferably sweet, as glucose in your bloodstream will make the baby more responsive.

The test can be performed either in your doctor's office or in the hospital. You will be asked to lie on your side on an examining couch or bed so that you can be linked to a monitor that will pick up the fetal heart rate. A recorder is placed on your abdomen. When you feel the baby move, you press a button that makes a mark on the page.

The doctor is looking for what we call *fetal reactivity*, to ensure that the heart rate accelerates in association with an adequate number of movements. The test requires two or more fetal heart-rate accelerations of at least 15 beats per minute and 15 seconds duration in a 20-minute period.

The method is known as nonstress testing because it does not involve uterine contractions and the baby's movements are voluntary. The test can be repeated if necessary every three days.

Contraction stress testing (CST) is a refinement of the nonstress test technique. The test is performed if your doctor is concerned about the baby's health, and if the nonstress test has produced doubtful or suspicious results. Here, the doctor will intervene to stimulate uterine activity. The idea is to induce contractions but not labor. You will be closely monitored, and the fetal heart rate and contractions will be recorded. For the CST, you have to go to the hospital and have an intravenous infusion.

Again you will be asked to lie on a bed, with a monitor and recording device attached to your abdomen to trace the fetal heart rate and contractions. Pitocin will be administered through an intravenous line attached to your arm, which will cause contractions of the uterus.

Once you experience contractions at a rate of three contractions every 10 minutes, the doctor will watch to see that there is no drop in the baby's heart rate after each contraction. If there is a drop, then this may indicate an insufficient utero-placental reserve, that is, an inadequate supply of food and oxygen to the baby from the placenta. When the uterus contracts, it cuts off the supply of blood to the placenta and baby for those few seconds. If there is not enough glucose stored in the baby's heart to maintain a healthy heartbeat right through the contraction and afterward, then the baby has not been receiving sufficient nutrition. The pregnancy will then need further monitoring, or the baby may need to be delivered if the pregnancy is far enough along.

The Developing Science of Perinatology

Now, obstetricians are working even more closely with pediatricians, not only after the baby has been delivered but even before the birth. There are certain conditions that can be treated while the baby is still in the uterus; this is part of a brave new world called *perinatology*.

For example, the obstetrician may be able to diagnose a condition by removing blood from the umbilical cord and administering medication to the fetus by the same technique, while the baby is still in the uterus. This new relationship between obstetrician and pediatrician is the basis of perinatology, reflecting the fact that obstetric care and care of the newborn infant now overlap so closely.

Indeed, you may also have read about or seen on television the exciting new work from geneticists who are hoping to detect and treat, not just diagnose, inborn genetic problems. This type of "gene treatment" will always be controversial, because the procedure allows parents the opportunity to abort a fetus in situations where correction of the genetic problem is impossible. Only permitted for couples known to be carriers of problem genes, the test determines which embryo is clear of the inbred problem by locating genes for disorders such as cystic fibrosis, muscular dystrophy, and hemophilia. The scientists' aim is to help those couples afraid to give birth to a child to be able to have a healthy baby. They are basically preventing future terminations by couples who conceive, but then must wait for the results of the amniocentesis to determine genetic abnormality, and may have to make a decision whether to terminate a pregnancy at about 20 weeks.

Parents carrying the gene for a congenital condition may also have had to watch while a much-loved child slowly died of an inherited disease, or they may have witnessed a relative suffer. They may not be prepared to bring a child into this life who is so afflicted. So, although to some the technique may have the ring of parents shopping for the perfect baby, only parents known to have specific gene disorders are eligible for gene testing and, maybe one day, for gene manipulation.

How Do Scientists Spot Disorders
Caused by Gene Abnormalities?

The same method is used as for in vitro fertilization. The mother's eggs are collected after her ovaries have been stimulated to produce more than usual. On average, six eggs can be successfully fertilized. The scientists then clip off one or two cells on the third day after fertilization, when the beginning of a human life is a total of eight developing and multiplying cells. The size of this conceptus is smaller than the period at the end of this sentence.

By carrying out a cell biopsy, and then using genetic amplification techniques so that the cells multiply 3 to 4 million times, scientists can pinpoint certain inherited diseases. Some disorders might even be curable at this early stage, by insertion of a healthy gene into the fertilized eggs. Those deemed viable will then be replaced in the mother's womb. Under present regulations, this work has to be carried out before the embryo reaches 14 days, at which point the cells that eventually make up the baby organize themselves along a line called "the primitive streak."

No physician or scientist can predict who will be born with a genetic predisposition for diabetes or Alzheimer's disease by examining a single cell. But the technology to do so may also be just around the corner. There are, indeed, many exciting new technological advancements within the reproductive field, especially in early pregnancy. Now that we have a greater understanding of how fertilization occurs—and, more importantly, what goes wrong in that carefully laid-out plan—with subtle intervention we may one day be able to bring about changes to alleviate tragedy and the suffering of the newborn infant.

PART TWO

Why Did It Happen?
What Tests and Treatments
Are Available?

3

❦

What Are the Genetic Causes of a Miscarriage?

Chromosomal damage to the fetus? The thought preys heavily on the average parent's mind after the loss of a baby through a miscarriage. Most couples assume that the spontaneously lost baby was somehow malformed. Some people find they have recurrent dreams or nightmares that the baby was a kind of monster. Miscarriage is indeed commonly thought of as nature's quality control over babies not perfect enough to be born.

There has been a misunderstanding here, at least for those unfortunate couples who have miscarried several times. Chromosomal damage is very likely to be the cause of a *first, isolated miscarriage,* one that happens before the 12th week. Indeed, up to 50 percent of first, early miscarriages are known to be caused by such problems. But a second or third miscarriage is less likely to be chromosomally abnormal, especially if prior losses tested normally. The literature is conflicting on the subject for many reasons, as the studies have been confined to only very early miscarriages or are retrospective in nature. Chromosomal abnormalities are not necessarily a recurring problem; indeed, their incidence becomes less with recurrent losses, and their contribution to repeated losses is small.

If you miscarry, genetic testing must be done to determine the cause of your miscarriages. If your doctor finds you have miscarried and the pregnancy is still inside you, then it must be removed as soon as possible. This is usually performed by suction in your doctor's office. The pregnancy tissue will be sent to a genetics laboratory for analysis of the chromosomes. The fresher the tissue, the greater the chance that the laboratory will be able to grow the cells and see if there is a chromosomal abnormality.

If you miscarry at home, you should try to collect the embryonic or pregnancy tissue (which is grayish in appearance, as compared to the deep red of the blood clots). Although this may seem upsetting or traumatic, the results are worth the effort. Place the material in a clean container, if possible in a sterile saline solution (such as that for contact lenses) in the refrigerator, but not in the freezer. Take it to your doctor the next morning so it can be sent to the appropriate laboratory.

The results of such tests can take from two to six weeks to come through. If they are abnormal, you will have the reassurance that this was the cause of that miscarriage and further investigations will not be necessary. It is also not likely to recur.

If this is not your first miscarriage, ask your doctor to do the genetic testing. Even if it is your first pregnancy loss, and you are over 35, have suffered infertility or have become pregnant using IVF (or a similar procedure), then it should be done, too.

What Makes Chromosomal Problems Happen?

Advanced maternal age is the best-known cause of chromosomally based miscarriages. Why this is so is not fully understood. But as I mentioned in Chapter 2, the mother's eggs may be showing the effects of age, which can cause abnormalities in cell division. It is interesting to note that more early miscarriages are of female than of male embryos, for reasons no one knows.

Problems usually occur spontaneously during the tenuous process of fertilization and the ensuing miraculous fusion of sperm and egg, which manage to combine to make one new human being.

When fertilization happens, an egg is usually fertilized by one sperm in the fallopian tube. It all sounds so simple, but, in fact, it is very complicated. Before conception, the chromosomes of the egg and sperm cells must first divide (*meiosis*), so that each contains only 23 chromosomes (half the number for a human being). Then when they join, they will have the normal chromosome number, 46. If problems occur during this process, chromosomal abnormalities may result, which in turn may lead to a miscarriage.

Suppose your doctor has recommended that you and your partner attend genetic counseling, or the material from your miscarriage was sent to a genetics laboratory for chromosome testing. Just what information is your doctor looking for?

The Lives of Chromosomes and Genes

Our bodies are constructed of millions of cells, living, dying, changing all the time. Some cells live for a few months, others for years. A woman's egg cells, for example, can live for 45 to 50 years. All of these body cells contain chromosomes, which are long threadlike structures that operate in pairs and look something like two arms. The genes, containing the DNA code that imprints physical characteristics such as the color of our hair and eyes, our blood type, and even our personalities, comprise hundreds of minuscule dots on the chromosomes.

Unlike the genes, the chromosomes are distinguishable under the microscope. Back in the 1880s, it was discovered that these threadlike structures can absorb a special kind of dye and so become visible. (Their name derives from the Greek words *chroma,* meaning color, and *soma,* meaning body.) Although we now use highly sophisticated techniques to view the chromosomes, the basis remains the same. The chromosomes are stained and investigated under magnification. The pairs are assessed for the right number, the proper structure, and the possibility of damage to individual ones.

Each of us has 46 chromosomes in every cell: 23 of our chromosomes were inherited from our mother and the other 23 from our father, including one sex chromosome from each parent. If we inherit an X and a Y chromosome, we became male; two X chromosomes and we became female (see Figure 4).

So each individual has 22 pairs, known as autosomes, plus two sex chromosomes (XX or XY), totaling to the requisite 46. During meiosis, which occurs just before the moment of conception, each cell has only 22 autosomes plus 1 sex chromosome, so that when the sperm and egg lock sides, they will create one complete whole. When romantics write of falling in love and talk about finding the "other half" to your whole, they are indeed quite right!

Random selection decides which two cells, with particular genes attached to the chromosomes, will meet and mate. This is

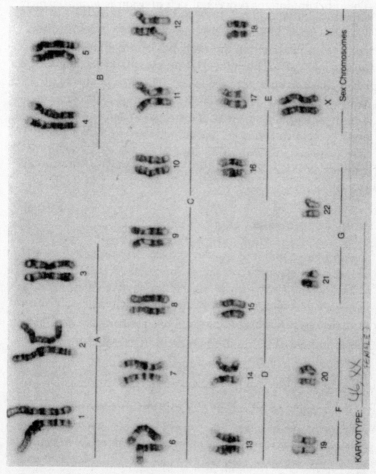

Figure 4. Photo of normal chromosome content of a human cell, obtained through amniocentesis.

also why we are all unique. Genetic features, therefore, are set in motion from that moment of fertilization when the different genes meet and match.

The other important process of cell division is *mitosis,* which takes place within 12 to 24 hours after the egg and sperm have met. This process marks the beginning of rampant cell multiplication as the conceptus begins to grow. At this stage some chromosomes can be lost or broken. If an extra chromosome called a *trisomy* is present, this may lead to deformities. For example, an extra chromosome 21 is the cause of Down syndrome. Embryos with these kinds of abnormalities usually miscarry early, and as I have emphasized before, such miscarriages usually do not occur again.

What Abnormalities Might Occur?

In a very small number of couples with repeat miscarriages—only about 3 to 5 percent—one or both partners may in fact have an abnormality in *their* chromosomes. This abnormality may have no affect on their own lives but may affect the fetus. For example, an abnormality in your chromosomes may not be reflected in your appearance, but if it affects the number of chromosomes in your egg cell, then it could cause a problem when meiosis takes place.

A patient of mine had a certain rare malposition of her chromosomes. She was very upset to learn about this and needed a lot of reassurance that she was absolutely normal—not a freak. However, the only way the couple could try for a normal baby, unfortunately, was just to keep trying. They would possibly have to put up with repeated miscarriages until one conception managed to override the problem. Once that occurred, their chances of having a normal healthy baby were good. Sadly, in such a rare case, nothing can be done to prevent or treat the problem. At this time, there is no way we can alter the body's chromosomal makeup. Someday in the future, through work that is now being done with in vitro programs, it will be possible to extract genetic information from a fertilized egg and provide preventive treatment.

Similarly, another patient who was happily looking forward to her first baby at the age of 43 discovered after amniocentesis that the fetus had an extra set of chromosomes (69, instead of 46, called a *triplody*). She decided to terminate the pregnancy, as she knew it was unlikely to be a recurring problem (two sperm had entered one egg) and that she stood a good chance of a normal pregnancy the next time.

Translocation is a term you might come across in a discussion of chromosomes. With this condition, there is the correct number of chromosomes but the pieces are joined up incorrectly. We now know that 7 percent of couples with recurrent miscarriage have a translocation, but we cannot predict whether subsequent chromosomal abnormalities will occur in their children. You may have inherited this problem from one of your parents, but in your own conception it was balanced out. If a similar problem affects your partner, then it could be a cause of recurrent miscarriages for you as a couple. It is a rare condition but one that can be tested for.

When Should You Go for Genetic Counseling?

If testing of a miscarriage specimen reveals abnormal chromosomes, your doctor may recommend genetic counseling and you would be advised to have an amniocentesis or chorionic villus sampling (both are discussed later in this chapter) in the next pregnancy to ensure the absence of chromosomal disorders in the fetus. Obviously the ideal situation would be to prevent chromosomal abnormalities occurring in the first place, but this is not yet possible.

You should also consider genetic counseling, because of the chromosomal effects of aging, if you are over 35 or if there is a history of a gene disorder such as cystic fibrosis or Tay-Sachs disease in your family. Fortunately, such disorders are rare, but in many cases it is now possible to test for them.

Similarly, if you have previously given birth to a child with a congenital abnormality, even if the child was from a previous marriage, or if as a couple you are in any way related, you should seek counseling to assess the risk of recurrence.

What Happens at Genetic Counseling?

The counselor will ask you many questions about your families, going back as far as three generations. You will be asked medical details about any branch of either family—the number of miscarriages, stillbirths, and children who died in infancy. Free forms, called family medical records, can be obtained from the March of Dimes, so that you can begin working on them at home in preparation for the genetic history.

If there are indications for further investigation, blood will be drawn from you and your partner and sent to a laboratory to check your chromosomes. The results will take a few days to arrive, as your white blood cells have to be grown in the laboratory. Once the cells begin to divide and multiply, the process of mitosis, they are compressed, and the chromosomes are spread out, identified, and matched into pairs to see if they are normal.

Fetal Chromosome Testing

Chromosome testing on the fetus can also be done while you are pregnant via several techniques.

Pre-implantation Genetic Diagnosis (PGD)

This technique may be an alternative to later testing of the fetus during pregnancy. Embryos, fertilized eggs obtained through IVF, are tested before being inserted back into the mother's womb. The advantage is that abnormal embryos won't be inserted for implantation so the pregnancy won't be threatened. The main indication for this test, which is expensive, is that the mother is over 35. PGD does not detect all abnormalities, but it does include the more common ones, including Down syndrome. The test takes about eight hours, and any embryo which is seen to be normal can then be transferred to the womb. PGD is not available in all IVF centers, so if you are concerned about whether you will need PGD, discuss this issue with your doctor. This procedure is important in that it will help improve the success rate of IVF, eradicating some of the underlying causes for IVF failure.

Amniocentesis

If you are already pregnant, the geneticist can work with fetal cells found in the amniotic fluid. Amniocentesis is the name given to the process of extraction of amniotic fluid for chromosomal analysis, or genetics testing, on the baby. This is usually performed from the 16th week of pregnancy, when there is sufficient amniotic fluid to make its removal safe. An ultrasound is done first to locate the fetus, placenta, and pool of fluid. The doctor then inserts a hollow needle through your abdominal wall, and the amniotic fluid is drawn up through the needle into a vial. It usually takes 10 working days to obtain the results, while the cells are grown and the chromosomes are analyzed.

It can be alarming for the pregnant woman, already entering her 5th month, to watch the long needle invading her abdomen and to worry about whether this will cause a miscarriage. Surprisingly, the procedure is not at all painful. Amniocentesis does carry a small further risk of miscarriage, but this has lessened over the years as doctors become more and more skilled in the procedure and the use of ultrasound. The risk of a miscarriage can run from 1 in 200 to 1 in 400, with a doctor who performs amniocentesis frequently. If you are going to be 35 or over by the time of the baby's birth, then the risk-benefit factor may justify its use.

Chorionic Villus Sampling (CVS)

Fetal cells for study can also be obtained by this technique, which is done earlier in pregnancy than amniocentesis. Usually from week 11 on (but not before), a small sample of placental tissue is taken from the pregnancy and analyzed. A tube is inserted through the cervix or sometimes through the abdomen into the womb. Results are available in 10 working days. The advantage of CVS is that it can be performed earlier in pregnancy, so that if a serious chromosomal defect is discovered, a termination can be performed earlier if decided upon.

The disadvantage of CVS is that it carries a slightly higher risk of miscarriage than amniocentesis, around 1 in 100. It is therefore worth going to a center where the procedure is done routinely to minimize this risk. Further, with CVS, confusion may arise in interpreting the results if there is a mixture of chromosome karyotypes (or patterns) in the rapidly growing placental cells.

If you have experienced an early miscarriage, it would be important to learn whether its cause *was* chromosomal. You would then not need to take all the other tests to discover the possible causes of your miscarriage. Coupled with the fact that a major chromosomal problem in both parents is very rare, the news should make your next attempt at pregnancy a much less anxious time.

Since both amniocentesis and CVS carry a risk of miscarriage, couples who have already suffered several pregnancy losses or infertility may find that putting their next pregnancy at further risk is unacceptable. You and your partner will have to discuss very carefully with each other and with your doctor the value of the tests and their side effects. However, medicine's attempt to develop a nonrisky and noninvasive way of testing for chromosome abnormalities has resulted in much ongoing research to develop new procedures that won't have a risk of pregnancy loss, such as the tests described here that are already available.

Nuchal Translucency

This first-trimester screening technique for chromosomal abnormalities including Down syndrome is gaining ground in medical circles. An ultrasound measurement of abnormally increased nuchal translucency (an echo-free area at the back of the fetal neck) is done. At the same time, the mother's blood is tested for the presence of two proteins that would also be indicators of an abnormality.

The ultrasound must be done before 13 weeks 6 days—ideally at 11 weeks. The test is only about 90 percent accurate, but it may guide couples in their decision making. If it reveals an increased risk for a chromosome problem, it could lead to a decision to go ahead with CVS or later with amniocentesis. If you are under 35, it can also be worth having the sonogram for extra reassurance.

Alpha-Fetoprotein (AFP)

This is a test done on a sample of the mother's blood after week 16 of the pregnancy (the second trimester). It is now a routine part of pregnancy care in the United States and in other industrialized countries, and if elevated it helps diagnose neural tube (brain and spinal cord) defects such as spina bifida. Along with the AFP, other hormones are also measured, including human chorionic gonadotrophin (HCG) and estriol. They are produced by the fetus and are passed into the mother's bloodstream, which is why the tests can be done on her blood.

A *low* AFP, however, suggests a chromosomal problem such as Down syndrome and an amniocentesis would then be done.

Routine Ethnic Genetic Blood Screening

Every pregnant couple, or even those planning a pregnancy, will be screened as part of the prenatal visit for abnormal genes; which gene tests are done depends on the couple's history and ethnic background—for example, for disorders such as abnormal red blood cell proteins, cystic fibrosis, or Tay-Sachs disease. If the mother's blood test shows her to be an abnormal gene carrier, then her husband or partner will also need to be tested as these are recessive conditions. If he too shows the same abnormal gene, the couple will have a 1 in 4 chance of the baby being born with the condition. In such a situation, the mother can undergo an amniocentesis during pregnancy to see whether or not the fetus has the disease.

Fetal Blood Sampling

This involves taking a sample of the fetus's blood from the umbilical cord, through a needle guided by ultrasound into the mother's abdomen. It is usually done after 18 weeks to check chromosomes—for example, if the fetus appears to be anatomically abnormal—or to rule out infection in the fetus.

As you will read in some of the accounts in this book, many women have had to make the difficult decision whether to have genetic testing. Very often, despite their reluctance to terminate a pregnancy after years of struggling to save one, they may have the chromosomal testing for reassurance and because of their fear of not being able ever to have a normal healthy child.

4

⨪

What Are the Anatomical Causes
of a Miscarriage?

In the previous chapters, I mentioned that an incompetent cervix is a very common cause of second-trimester miscarriages (those occurring sometime between the 13th to the 24th week). It is also now well known that congenital abnormalities (meaning those anomalies you are born with) of the uterus can cause second-trimester, and even in some cases, first-trimester, miscarriages. For these reasons, one of the major points of investigation will be checking the structure of your uterus and cervix.

The fallopian tubes, uterus, and upper portion of the vagina are all formed within the first 5 to 6 weeks following conception from two structures known as the *müllerian* and *wolffian* ducts. The müllerian ducts form the reproductive organs, and the wolffian ducts form the kidneys and urinary tract. Both are of vital importance in the developing female fetus. Between weeks 6 and

7 following conception, these ducts begin a process of change, during which problems may occur.

In week 9, the two müllerian ducts cross above the wolffian tract, where they fuse in the middle of the body to form a single cavity that will become the uterus and vagina. (In the male embryo, the same cavity will have degenerated by week 10.) The vagina does not open as a canal, however, until the 20th to the 22nd week. At any stage during this normal course of fusion something can go wrong.

Heredity may play a part in the abnormalities, or drugs such as DES taken by your mother could also be responsible. DES not only damaged the vagina in many female fetuses, but it led to a special form of uterine abnormality known as the *T-shaped uterus*.

The basic differences in uterine shapes are illustrated in Figure 5. In about 50 percent of cases the uterus is *bicornuate* or *septate*: a band extends down the middle of the uterus toward the cervix. The *didelphic uterus* has two separate cornua, or horns, and two separate cervices.

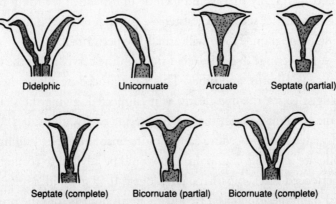

Figure 5. Some of the uterine abnormalities that can occur.
In the middle of the lower row is one of the more common
abnormalities found.

Some of the more common abnormalities may have been caused by one or both of the müllerian ducts failing to develop, leading to an absence of one-half of the uterus. Or the ducts may have failed to fuse, leaving uterine structures without proper cavities.

Such abnormalities of the uterus are more common than doctors used to think. Studies performed on women who are evaluated for infertility show congenital abnormalities of the uterus as frequently as 1 percent to 10 percent of this population. However, in a study of women sterilized through the cervix, the incidence was 1.9 percent. This latter figure is probably more typical for the general population, in that this was a group of women not experiencing trouble conceiving. Nevertheless, a statistic of nearly 2 percent is still a very high one.

How Are These Anomalies Diagnosed?

If your doctor feels that your history indicates structural defects—typically that would include unexplained recurrent miscarriages in the second trimester—a procedure known as a hysterosalpingogram (HSG) will usually be performed.

A radiopaque dye is injected through the cervix to fill the cervical canal, uterus, and tubes. This x-ray procedure allows the radiologist to see the dye clearly as it is injected, giving the shapes of the relevant parts in the cervix, uterine cavity, and tubes. Unfortunately, the procedure can be quite uncomfortable, leading to moderate to severe cramping. You would be advised to request an experienced and sympathetic radiologist. It's a good idea to take a mild painkiller, such as Tylenol, about an hour before the procedure. You may also be given antibiotics before and after the procedure to avoid any risk of infection from the dye. You should try to arrange the date of the procedure for just after a period to make sure you are not pregnant.

An excellent new technique using safe ultrasound (no x-rays), done either by your gynecologist or a radiologist, checks the inside of the womb to see that it is normal and that there is no scar tissue or polyps. This is called *sonohysterography* or *saline sonogram*. The doctor uses a vaginal ultrasound probe. Before insertion, a small amount of sterile saline is injected through the cervix into the uterine cavity, allowing this potential space to be imaged. The procedure is accurate, comfortable, safe, and noninvasive.

Hysteroscopy is a technique that also provides visual examination of your uterus. A special fiber-optic hysteroscope is inserted into the vagina and cervix. For this procedure, the cervix is dilated, using a cervical block or general anesthetic, and the uterus is inspected along all its walls to look for abnormalities such as polyps, congenital bands, or adhesions (scarring). These can be treated at the same time, through the hysteroscope, making it a very helpful test.

Laparoscopy is another method for inspecting the uterus and fallopian tubes. A laparoscope is inserted through the umbilicus (belly button). Prior to insertion of the laparoscope, your stomach is filled with carbon dioxide gas. The laparoscope is used for direct visual examination to support a diagnosis. You will be brought into the hospital for a day, as the procedure is performed under a general anesthetic.

Using a laparoscope the doctor can see whether there is a double or partially split uterus, or adhesions binding the fallopian tubes. The doctor will also check for endometriosis, a condition in which some of the uterine lining (endometrium) grows outside the uterus in the pelvic area, causing fertility problems. Dye is injected to see if it spills readily through the tubes. Your appendix will also be checked to see whether it is healthy. Following the procedure, you will have a few stitches in the umbilicus and possibly in your lower abdomen near your pubic region where a probe or probes may have been placed. The stitches will not need to be removed because they usually dissolve on their own.

These types of investigations once would only have been performed on women with infertility problems. But now, more and more, they are being used on women with a history of miscarriage.

Hysteroscopic resection is the procedure that corrects uterine deformities from inside the uterus. It is performed with the help of a hysteroscope and may avoid the need for abdominal surgery to correct the shape of the uterus (known as *metroplasty*). As with any form of abdominal surgery, this would not only have involved general anesthesia and a lengthy recovery time, but also the uterus would be surgically opened up, and this could lead to problems in a future pregnancy.

Following corrective surgery on the uterus, the success rate for a healthy birth is about 80 percent. But, as ever, the advantages of surgical techniques have to be weighed against possible risks. Surgery may cause scarring of the uterus, which could affect fertility. Where surgery is not required to correct a congenital abnormality of the uterus, treatment may range from doing nothing, to removing a polyp (a little piece of tissue) or scarring, to placing a suture in the cervix when you next become pregnant.

There is a simple test for an incompetent cervix, often done in the doctor's office, whereby metal dilators are passed gently into the cervix. If they pass easily, the cervix is deemed weak.

Other Uterine Problems That May
Need Correction

Intrauterine Adhesions

Hysteroscopy and hysterograms may reveal that you have *intrauterine adhesions*, or scarring inside the womb. Patients often find it difficult to visualize such a problem. Basically, these adhesions are pieces of scar tissue, or bands, that crisscross the lining of the womb (endometrium) like a spider's web from one side wall to another. They have long been identified as a cause of fertility problems. We now know they may play a role in miscarriages, too.

In extreme cases, the entire uterine cavity is obliterated and menstruation may cease. This is called Asherman's syndrome and was reported as far back as the end of the nineteenth century. For other women, the scars mean there is insufficient lining of the womb for the embryo to grow healthily.

The scars may be caused by intrauterine infection, D&C procedures (such as is required following a miscarriage), or from late elective abortions (terminations). They occur in as many as 15 percent of women who have had a D&C after a pregnancy condition but are rare in women having a D&C unassociated with such a condition.

Once diagnosed by a hysterogram, the scars can be excised by dilating the cervix under general anesthesia and then cutting through the adhesions. This is done with the use of the hysteroscope, which makes each adhesion visible before cutting. An IUD (intrauterine device) is then placed in the uterus, and the patient is put on a course of estrogen, which prevents the adhesions from reforming. Once treated, the patient is advised to try for a pregnancy as quickly as possible.

Fibroids

Fibroids (or fibromyomas) are benign tumors of the muscle and fibrous tissue of the uterine wall. They can be present at different locations in the wall of the uterus: either in the thick middle section of the wall, where they are called intramural; on the surface of the uterus, where they are called subserous (and in this position they can also be on long stalks or *pedunculated* and feel separate from the uterus); or in the depth of the uterine wall and bulging into the uterine cavity, where they are called submucus.

By the age of 40, about 40 percent of women have fibroids. Remember that they are benign swellings and generally do not require any treatment whatsoever unless they have grown very large in a short space of time or they cause severe bleeding or pressure in the pelvis. Their role in causing miscarriages has been exaggerated; they are, in fact, an unusual cause of a miscarriage. Even during a continuing pregnancy, they seldom give any problem, except for some pain if they grow too large for their blood supply and soften. They may rarely cause premature labor if the placenta happens to implant over a fibroid. In general, fibroids, and certainly the small ones, should not be removed surgically in an effort to prevent miscarriage. They are best left alone.

Are Uterine Abnormalities a Common Cause of Miscarriage?

Abnormalities of the uterus may be responsible for a wide variety of gynecologic disorders, from infertility to miscarriage to premature labor or hemorrhage following delivery. Or they may cause none of the above. The medical literature shows that uterine abnormalities account for up to 12 percent of recurrent miscarriages, particularly those that take place between 12 and 24 weeks. Some women with an incompetent cervix may also have an abnormal uterus. Yet surprisingly, considering the extent of some abnormalities, that figure is not high. To look at the figures another way, the majority of women with uterine abnormalities will not experience any reproductive problem. However, an incompetent cervix is one abnormality that must be treated early in pregnancy as it has a very high risk of causing a late miscarriage.

Sophia had a history of an incompetent cervix. After long and agonizing years of infertility and the loss of a baby in midpregnancy, there is a happy ending for Sophia and her husband, who now have two delightful children.

My Cervix Was So Effaced That I Could See My Daughter's Hand Reaching into the Cervical Canal

Sophia is in her midforties. Charming, beautiful, highly intelligent, and creative, she had her first child, a son, with no problems at all. She conceived two days after getting married at age 38. During that pregnancy she swam, exercised, and walked in the hills. The birth was vaginal, in a birthing center, all very normal. Since that easy first experience of pregnancy and birth, however, it's been a very different story.

❦

The most dramatic problem was when I began to lose a baby after an amniocentesis. I'd had previous early miscarriages, but on this occasion I agreed to have the amnio test because of my age. Two days later, I went to the bathroom and saw the entire amniotic sac coming out. It was the most terrifying experience of my life. I pushed it back and went to lie down with my feet up. This was in the middle of the night. We had to make a decision what to do. The doctor warned that there was a serious risk of infection. We were living in upstate New York at the time. In the end, we agreed to an induced labor and that the baby would not survive. There were just too many risks involved. I had a stillbirth. The baby was alive until the moment of birth. I was lying there on morphine and they brought the dead fetus for me to hold. They took pictures and asked me what I wanted to do with it. That was such a tragic, painful, traumatic experience; I find it hard to talk about still.

I had no idea whether the stillbirth was brought on by the amnio or whether I had an incompetent cervix. So when I was pregnant the next time, I changed doctors and the new doctor was very sympathetic. He agreed that I'd never want to do amniocentesis or CVS, but we could tell a lot about the fetal condition by high resolution sonogram. I had one at 16 weeks and then again at 20 weeks. At that point, my cervix was beginning to efface. The baby was fine, but I was sent home to do bed rest and was put on medication to slow down contractions. I stayed at my mother-in-law's house, which is close to the city.

At that time my son was 4 years old. We were still living upstate and were about to move. My husband and son went back, but I stayed to be near the doctor and hospital. The next day, I got up and went to the doctor's office for one more sonogram to reassure me. That's when we saw that the cervix was really effaced. On the screen, I saw my daughter's hand reaching into the cervical canal. She was asking me to save her. I went immediately to the hospital. I was hooked up on medication to slow contractions. My only chance was to have a stitch put in. At 22 weeks, that carries a 25 percent chance of miscarriage, but there was no choice.

The doctor put a double stitch in—tied through a sterile flat button (to anchor the stitch more firmly)—that's his speciality! I was in intensive care for 10 days, on antibiotics. Then I was moved to a regular maternity ward, where I spent the next three months with my feet raised above my head. Total bed rest. I didn't get up to go to the bathroom or anything. How do you get through it? Every week, another milestone would be reached. Each one was a sort of victory. I read a lot, talked on the phone. My computer broke so I even gave up on that. I'd have breakfast late and then concentrate on relaxation techniques, exercising in bed, and massage. You look forward to visitors. I even had my high school reunion around my hospital bed. When my son, who hadn't seen me for three weeks, came to visit, he crawled into my bed and stayed there for eight hours. The experience was good for him and my husband. They learned to bond and coped without me.

I got such wonderful care. In some ways, it was the best three months of my life. I was incubating the fetus and they were incubating me. The hospital was like a womb. I was so well taken care of. My doctor would come to visit and he gave me such hope. He also is a very intuitive doctor and did not just go by the book. He decided against all invasive measures. We just stuck to the bed rest and let gravity do its work.

At 28 weeks, that's another time for celebration, as the baby could likely survive if born. At 34 weeks, I was discharged and had to practice walking. I was scared to be up and outside. It was August 18 and I remember thinking "I missed the whole summer." I went to my parents' house and straight back to bed. I only walked a little. At 37 weeks, I got out of bed. They took the stitch out and told me to take a jog in Central Park! In fact, she wasn't born until the 39th week, when my water finally broke. She was born quickly by vaginal delivery, weighing 6 pounds. I'm going to have the button from the stitch procedure made into a necklace for her. This was not merely high-risk pregnancy care; this was all a miracle!

"There Were Times I Was So Depressed That I Couldn't Get Out of Bed"

Kori is a lovely, big-hearted woman of 41, with twins who are now 9 years old. When we met in early summer, she brought the boy with her because he was off school, having been sick all night. The girl was at school. Kori is a very emotional woman. Just talking about her experiences brought her to tears as we spoke.

I had two years' worth of miscarriages—five in all. They started when I was age 29. When I got married, I just assumed I'd be a mother by 30. But it was the most awful period of my life. The miscarriages were all very early, before even a heartbeat could be seen. They were just empty sacs—known as blighted ova. The terms upset me even more. There were times I was so depressed that I couldn't get out of bed. I was in such a state. In other couples, all that misery and failure could have led to divorce. But, fortunately, my husband and I are such good friends. All I ever wanted was to have a child. But I was beginning to lose my faith in life.

I was with a regular doctor and everyone said it was all normal. But even after the second miscarriage, I wanted to move on. I took myself to a fertility endocrinologist. He worked on the assumption that maybe my eggs weren't strong enough, because I obviously had no problem conceiving. But during ovulation, I always produced good eggs. After two more losses, we had some immune therapy treatment. I conceived but lost that pregnancy, too. At this point, it was recommended that either I adopt or find an egg donor—because I would never have my own child. I'd gone as far as finding a friend who might be the egg donor. Then I came across the book *Preventing Miscarriage.* Even though it meant waiting three months for an appointment with the author, I booked myself in.

When we met, the new doctor told my husband and me that we should be able to have our own baby. We both came out of that meeting in tears. There were three different tests he ordered that no one else had done. First, they found an infection in my husband's sperm, and he was given an antibiotic for that. Second, even though I was ovulating and conceiving, they did a test on the lining of the womb. Third, it was found that my anticardiolipin antibodies were raised. I was put on prednisone, a steroid, to lower the antibodies. Although I was only 31, I felt old with such a history.

But the doctor told me to relax and take a warm bath when I was ovulating. We did conceive without help. I was on the prednisone, we saw the heartbeats. We really were hoping for twins, as they do run in the family, and sure enough, there were two heartbeats. I was so happy, at last! But, unfortunately, after that sonogram, I had bad bleeding for the whole of the first trimester. Not just staining, but really bad bleeding. It was really scary. It seems this is common with twin pregnancies, but I was terrified that the bleeding might get worse. I was also on progesterone suppositories. I went to see my doctor every week for the first 13 weeks—then every other week. I had blood work and sonograms all the time. I felt very cared for.

One downside to the steroids is they bloat you up. I'm only 5 feet tall and with twins, heavy, bloated, losing all that blood—I can tell you I wasn't a pretty sight!

I also have a bicornuate uterus. The doctor was concerned that I might go only to the 8th month, as the uterus might not be big enough for twins. So I also had to have a cerclage stitch to close my cervix. The day it was scheduled for, I had some bleeding, but they did the procedure anyway. Everyone was very aware that I might have problems later in the pregnancy. Surprisingly, my water broke at 35 weeks. I had a C-section with the stitch still in and the twins were born. My daughter was 3 pounds 5 ounces and my son was 4 pounds. They both had very strong lungs, probably due to the prednisone I'd been taking. The night they were born, I was actually monitoring my contractions when the water broke.

By that time, I was also on bed rest. But I was so huge and short of breath that I wasn't exactly up to doing much. I used to wonder sometimes how I'd get across a road! I was so grateful, I really tried hard not to complain.

I'm so thankful to have had children. I'd suffered so much and just can't get over the fact I had my own lovely twins. I tell friends, "If I can have children, so can you. Don't give up hope." It's amazing how many women have called me to discuss their issues. People either pass on my phone number or they hear about me. I always give them my support. I've even had other women send me their baby pictures!

❦

What Makes an Incompetent Cervix?

Losing a baby in the second trimester can be a devastating experience, as we read in Philippa's story in Chapter 1. One of the especially sad facts about cervical incompetence is that these women have been losing pregnancies regularly, often at the same week in each pregnancy. Not only is any miscarriage a harrowing experience, but to find yourself repeatedly losing healthy, normal babies—who, if you could see or hold them, look like miniature newborns—can lead a woman, and her partner, to despair. Later in this chapter we will hear the story of Lisa, who has indeed gone through just this type of experience. This is unfortunately a fairly common problem. But with new techniques, we can now offer much more hope for successful treatment.

The actual incidence of incompetent cervix is unknown but is thought to be about 1 to 2 percent of normal deliveries. It has been estimated that an incompetent cervix is the cause of up to one-fifth of late miscarriages (that is, those following the 12th week).

Technically speaking, a cervix is classified as incompetent if it fails to maintain an intrauterine pregnancy to term. The cervix begins to dilate far too early and easily, the amniotic membranes push through, and, following either a dramatic rupture of the membranes or blood loss, the woman go into a rapid, short premature labor. The baby is then born too early for independent life. Although the procedure of inserting a stitch to hold the cervix closed has been in practice since 1951, only recently have doctors fully understood just what can happen to the cervix. We are now better able to diagnose and treat the condition successfully.

Normally, the cervix acts as the plug that holds the pregnancy in place. The cervix is mainly composed of collagen, or connective tissue, and only 10 percent of it is muscle. When you are not pregnant the cervix is rigid, fibrous, and hard. But it softens during late pregnancy, an action known as "ripening" that is probably caused by the action of the pregnancy hormones. If the cervix ripens too early, the pregnancy can be pushed through a weakened cervix from about the 14th to the 20th week.

All too often the cervix has been affected prior to the pregnancy by trauma—for example, from previous D&Cs or elective terminations of pregnancy. Until recently no one realized how gingerly the cervix should be treated. For example, one method of treatment for painful periods used to be dilating, or overstretching, the cervix, which usually tore the muscle fibers and led to incompetence. This treatment is now unnecessary because of the availability of effective medication for menstrual pain. In addition, with our increased medical knowledge, there is no reason why induced abortions (terminations) should now result in incompetent cervix.

If an abortion is needed after the 10th or 11th week, when the cervix would otherwise have to be dilated, your doctor does not have to use metal dilators, which can tear and damage the cervix. Instead, the cervix can be ripened, or softened, using laminaria sticks, which are inserted into the cervix and left overnight before the procedure. In addition, a hormone called prostaglandin is inserted into the vagina either as a tablet, a suppository, or a cream, which also helps to soften the cervix. The risks of mechanical trauma and damage to the cervix can thus be obviated.

The cervix can unfortunately also be damaged in childbirth, torn either by the passage of the infant during delivery or by instruments such as forceps or a vacuum extractor. The other major cause of an incompetent cervix, as we discussed earlier in the chapter, is uterine abnormalities, which, by preventing expansion of the top of the uterus as the pregnancy grows, force the cervix to open below.

A diagnosis of incompetent cervix can be made from a combination of the patient's reproductive history, which is most important, and an internal examination. Hysterography can also be used for diagnosis. The dye may spill back around the instrument that has been placed in the cervix and through which the dye is injected, to show the width of the cervix.

Serial ultrasounds of the pregnant cervix, in expert hands, have an important place for the diagnosis of an incompetent cervix. For example, if you are already pregnant you may be able to see on the screen a very short cervix (20 to 25 millimeters, compared to a normal cervix of about 35 to 40 millimeters). If the radiographer presses on the top of the womb, it may be possible to see the amniotic sac bulging down. Transvaginal ultrasound is very useful in diagnosing abnormalities of the cervix.

The main indication of a weak cervix is a past history of recurrent miscarriages between 14 and 24 weeks. Usually there will have been moderate bleeding; the membranes may even have ruptured before any contractions were felt. The contractions that do come are short and, though usually quite painless, may give a feeling of pressure. The fetus is often, very sadly, born alive.

Preventing Damage to the Cervix

Doctors treat D&C procedures with caution. They are aware that any woman in her reproductive years should not have her cervix forcibly dilated beyond Hegar 8 millimeters, to prevent tearing of the cervical fibers.

If you are in need of an advanced induced abortion, your doctor will probably ripen the cervix the night before, using laminaria or prostaglandins. This will greatly minimize the need for mechanical dilatation.

If you have an abnormal Pap smear that requires treatment, your doctor now has the option of using cryosurgery (freezing), laser therapy, or LEEP (where a small piece of the end of the cervix is removed), rather than surgical cone biopsy, in which a deeper portion of the cervix is cut away, possibly contributing to incompetence.

Why Does an Incompetent Cervix Give Way?

I have mentioned that the cervix is made up of only about 10 percent muscle; the rest of it is a fibrous material that can stretch and soften in pregnancy. The cervix opens at ovulation, allowing the entrance of sperm, but apart from that time it is normally closed.

During pregnancy, the cervix softens slightly, but otherwise it remains tightly closed to protect the fetus and uterine contents from the introduction of infection from the outside or the vagina. It is filled with a very thick or viscid mucus plug that stays in place until very late in pregnancy. At that point the cervix starts to shorten, or efface; it is beginning to open so the baby's head can go through it.

The part of the uterus above the cervix is made up mainly of strong muscle. During early pregnancy, the uterus increases in size due to pregnancy hormones, which cause muscle fibers in the body of the uterus to increase in number and to lengthen. Then, from the middle of the second trimester, from about 12 to 14 weeks on, the uterus also gets bigger because the growing fetus and amniotic sac now push up on the top of the uterus—the fundus—and cause its expansion. At around 40 weeks, the strong uterine muscle helps expel the baby through the cervical opening.

However, if the cervix is weak, or incompetent, or if the uterus is misshapen, this normal sequence of events does not occur. When there is a uterine abnormality, the muscle in the top of the uterus is often replaced by fibrous tissue that cannot expand. As the baby grows and pushes up on the fundus, the uterus refuses to give because of the fibrous tissue, and the pregnancy begins to act like a metal rod, pushing down on the cervix. This pressure begins around weeks 14 to 16. The membranes and amniotic sac are forced down into the weak cervix, which will start shortening and dilating. This will precipitate a rupture of the membranes, and a rapid miscarriage follows.

Symptoms are often very few. But if you do notice that your uterus is contracting and becoming very hard, if there is a very heavy mucus discharge or any vaginal bleeding, you should report to your doctor. Often no pain is experienced until the miscarriage is already well advanced. However, pressure on the cervix may produce a pain in the vagina that has been described as "like a knife pushing upward from the vagina into the pelvis." Severe backache may also occur. Any such symptoms around this time of pregnancy should be immediately reported.

However, if a diagnosis has been made and a stitch can be put in at the correct time, the success rate for producing a healthy term baby is very good, at least 80 to 90 percent. New studies have shown that the earlier in pregnancy the stitch is put in, and the higher up on the cervix your doctor can place it, the more effective is its hold. You and your doctor will be doing your best to simulate nature. The cervix needs to be closed and tight to maintain a pregnancy.

Sometimes an incompetent cervix, especially one that happens beyond about 20 weeks, may be associated with uterine contractions. It is not known whether this is true premature labor, or whether the weak cervix is causing the contractions. Nevertheless, at this late stage, in addition to the stitch, your doctor may put you on a drug such as Terbutaline to prevent further contractions. The drug is safe to take in pregnancy; its only side effect for you is a rapid heartbeat. It is approved for use after the 20th week of pregnancy.

How the Shirodkar or MacDonald Stitch Is Put In

The term *cerclage* can also be used to describe the procedure. It aptly describes the method whereby a stitch is placed around the cervix, making it much like a pouch where the strings have been pulled tight (see Figure 6). This famous technique is sometimes called a Shirodkar stitch, after one of its main proponents. Other doctors have lent their names to similar techniques, such as the MacDonald or Lash suture. These procedures are all modifications of cerelage.

A most important point to bear in mind is that the stitch should be put in early. It used to be said that it could not be

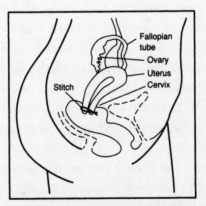

Figure 6. This diagram illustrates the placement of the cervical stitch.

placed before about week 14 because prior to the use of ultrasound, neither the doctor nor the patient would have heard the fetal heartbeat. Obviously, one would not want to put in a stitch if there was not a live pregnancy in the uterus. Now sonography can tell us if the fetus is alive from 6 weeks or even earlier.

I often recommend putting in the stitch around weeks 9 to 10. The earlier the stitch is in, the longer it may hold the pregnancy. One of the reasons is that while the cervix is still as long as it is going to be, it gives the doctor more to work with. And the stitch must always be placed as high up in the cervix as possible. Throughout pregnancy, the cervix normally contracts because it contains muscle tissue. This may cause the stitch to dislodge, and so it must be put in firmly.

If there are any overwhelming high-risk factors, and there is a question about the health of the fetus, chorionic villus sampling (CVS; see Chapter 3) can be done at week 11, prior to putting in the stitch.

Generally, the stitch should not be put in if you are actively bleeding or contracting, as the procedure may mask what is going to be an inevitable miscarriage and it won't help.

A stitch can even be placed in the cervix *before* you undertake a pregnancy. Usually this is only done where there is virtually no cervix present, making it technically very difficult or impossible to insert a stitch once the patient has become pregnant and the cervix has already begun to shorten. It is quite rare to do this, because putting a stitch in between pregnancies might interfere with fertility, and the technique used would almost inevitably mean a C-section delivery. As the timing and type of cerclage technique needed may vary from patient to patient, you must rely on your doctor's advice.

If your physician has decided that a stitch is needed, it will be done in the hospital. You will be admitted into the hospital on the day of the procedure. Some anesthesia will be necessary as the process is a little too painful otherwise. An epidural or spinal anesthetic, which is often used during labor, is a common choice. The procedure is done in the operating room. Your legs are placed in stirrups, and the technique usually takes about 15 to 30 minutes. Following the procedure you may be discharged on the same day or kept in the hospital overnight. The fetal heartbeat is checked afterward by ultrasound. The drug indomethacin is sometimes given to prevent contractions.

Treatment and Care After Surgery

You will be examined vaginally at each visit and also by ultrasound, to determine how secure the stitch is. If it has rolled down or if the cervix is beginning to open, your doctor may even decide to put in another stitch. Accidents can happen to the stitch itself: the knot may come loose, or the stitch can roll down the cervix and loosen. It is very important to see your doctor regularly, even once a week initially, until the fetus is viable at around 30 to 32 weeks.

As the stitch is a foreign body, it could be a site for infection. As a preventive measure, one week out of every month you may be prescribed an antibiotic, either by mouth or vaginally, to prevent infection. This is not always done and depends on the particular patient's history. I also take a culture or swab, from the stitch and cervix each month, to make sure there is no infection.

I have always believed in seeing patients with a history of miscarriage often and in giving a lot of reassurance. I believe this has a beneficial effect.

What If You Have Contractions
Even with the Stitch in Place?

Women needing a cervical stitch are often concerned about whether intercourse is safe or whether with a stitch it will set off contractions. If you feel comfortable about the idea and your doctor feels there is no inherent danger, you may be advised that it is safe to resume sexual intercourse. But you will probably be asked to use a condom to minimize infection and to avoid the possible effects of the prostaglandins from semen, which just might stimulate uterine contractions.

If premature labor does begin, it is treated vigorously with drugs such as Terbutaline and bed rest. Even with no signs of premature labor, if a patient is very high risk and anxious, I sometimes give her Terbutaline from 20 weeks.

When Is the Stitch Removed?

The stitch can be removed in the doctor's office and does not usually require hospitalization or an anesthetic. Removal is not painful. We aim for removal two weeks before the due date, at week 38. Once this stage is reached the baby is fully mature and the stitch can safely be removed.

We always try to remove the stitch before labor begins, because going into labor with the stitch in place could lead to a frantic rush to get it out in time for delivery. Delivery with the stitch in place could lead to tearing of the cervix. You also need a few days to allow any infection from the stitch site to leave your body.

After the stitch is removed, it is common to have minimal bright bleeding from the stitch site. Labor itself usually starts within hours or one to two days, especially if the cervix is very weak. However, labor may even be delayed *beyond* term in some cases, possibly because scarring from the stitch site helps hold the cervix closed!

The loss of a baby late in pregnancy can be so devastating that the mother or both parents can be left emotionally damaged. When Lisa and her husband came for a first appointment with their doctor, she was newly pregnant for the second time. They had just undergone the harrowing experience of losing their first baby, who was born at 25 weeks, weighing 1½ pounds. Lisa now has two children—a daughter in school and a little boy.

"He Weighed 1½ Pounds and They Were Keeping Him Alive in the Neonatal Intensive Care Unit."

❧

When I was 30, I got pregnant and at 20 weeks had to go to London for a two-week business trip. It never occurred to me that this might be a problem, as I was feeling so healthy and fit. I'd been there for two days when I started bleeding and cramping. I had had some cervical issues, but biopsies were taken and everything seemed fine. Well, there I was, trapped, a long way from home. I was bleeding a lot for days. But on a hospital visit, the sonogram showed the baby seemed fine. I went back to my hotel, but it all got worse. I was told to watch out for clotting.

Then I was brought onto the private hospital ward. I didn't realize that it's not so good to be in a private hospital in the UK, for high-risk conditions. They are not set up for emergencies. I was there for almost 5 weeks, still bleeding and cramping, My husband came to join me and in the end he had to give up his job to be able to stay with me. We went through all sorts of traumas. At one point, because they said the baby was about to be delivered, I had to be moved to an NHS [National Health Service] hospital, and the only one with a bed available was in the outer suburbs. In the end, he was born alive at 25 weeks. At first, he seemed to be in great shape. He weighed 1½ pounds and they were keeping him alive in the neonatal intensive care unit.

But then he began to go downhill. His lungs were not well formed and he stayed in the hospital for three months on a respirator. It was the most weird and awful time for us. We knew no one and lived in a small hotel near the hospital, spending all our days there. I don't think they took to us kindly in that hospital. They're not used to Americans being pushy and demanding new procedures. Later we were moved to a hospital in central London. I was there for another two months. Finally, one of the best U.S. doctors had us brought home in a private plane. The baby lived another month, before his heart finally gave out. It was a dreadful time, but by the time we lost him I had become pregnant again.

My new doctor guessed that the problem was with my cervix. He did a cerclage at 12 weeks and I stayed at home on bed rest. I walked a little at home, but never left the apartment except for those doctor visits once a week (which I so looked forward to). I was fortunate that my husband was still out of work, so he stayed home and looked after me the whole time. At 20 weeks, I was put on home monitoring, where they watch for contractions three to four times a day. It turned out to be a very good uneventful pregnancy. I was given medicine to relax the uterus. When the baby was mature, the doctor took the stitch out and still I didn't go into labor. In fact, I had to be induced after the due date. Everything was fine with the pregnancy and birth of my daughter.

With my next baby, I again had a stitch put in. My daughter was by then two years old and I was still working in my high-powered job. I wanted to work right through the pregnancy and was there for long hours. I saw my doctor every other week and worked right up to the due date. Again I was induced after the stitch was taken out. Now, our lives have reversed. My husband took an MBA during that time out of work. He has moved into a good career and I'm home with the children. The main thing is that we made it in the end. Right now, I'm content to stay home and take care of the children, after all we have been through.

❦

5

What Are the Hormonal Causes
of a Miscarriage?

Hormones take their name from the Greek word *horman,* meaning "to set in motion." They are the chemical messengers of the body, produced by tissues and organs. Some produce internal adjustments to the different systems of the body; others respond to external events and provoke behavioral reactions. As most women know from their menstrual cycle, our individual hormonal or endocrine balance contains very deep hidden clues to the functioning of our bodies.

Why some women's hormones are so imbalanced that they cannot sustain a pregnancy, we do not know. A surge in our understanding of the body's endocrinology occurred in 1973, when it was first learned how to measure actual sex hormone levels. Once the structure of hormones could be determined, it was possible even to offer hormone substitutes that have a similar effect on the body, to enhance the body's own natural hormones.

In the women's stories so far quoted, you have read of suppositories made of the most important hormone in early pregnancy, progesterone, used to help support the pregnancy. Later in this chapter, I will go more fully into the mysterious dance of life that is the reproductive cycle. For now, let us look at the explanation for hormone deficiency that, some believe, affects 10 to 15 percent of the women who miscarry. That is a sizable number of women.

Hormone Deficiency in Early Pregnancy

Progesterone is secreted by the corpus luteum, a little yellow cystic structure that appears on the ovary at midcycle after ovulation. Progesterone probably has many functions in addition to its importance in preparing the lining of the uterus to sustain the embryo. It has recently been shown that progesterone encourages implantation of the fertilized egg by regulating the mother's immune response to accept the foreign embryo (foreign to the mother's body because of the father's contribution). Another new theory is that progesterone acts against prostaglandin, which is a hormone that can cause inflammation and may be associated with miscarriage. Indeed, a lack of progesterone may lead to the embryo's miscarrying.

The corpus luteum in the ovary must keep up this work of providing nutrition and support for the embryo until the developing placenta can take over. The transition (also known as the luteo-placental shift) might take place any time from week 7 to week 10 of pregnancy. In effect, that means it starts to happen at about the 5th week following conception (pregnancy is always dated medically from the first day of your last period).

The corpus luteum lives only for about 10 weeks after ovulation (and conception). So, if a pregnancy is lost *before* week 10, it should be assessed for hormonal deficiency.

How can your doctor tell if you are suffering from a corpus luteum deficiency (CLD), also known as a luteal-phase defect (LPD)? If you experience pain at the time of ovulation (called the mittelschmertz), that means you are ovulating (producing an egg), and in effect you are also forming the corpus luteum. The pain is usually felt on one or both sides, low down in the abdomen. It lasts a few hours and is cramplike in nature. The pain may be accompanied by a sticky discharge that can even be blood-tinged. This is called an ovulation cascade. Note: The absence of such a discharge does *not* mean you are not ovulating.) If your temperature fails to rise during your normal menstrual cycle, this can be one signal of a corpus-luteum deficiency. The progesterone produced by the corpus luteum causes a temperature rise that lasts 10 to 14 days following ovulation. This thermal shift is measured with a special ovulation thermometer, not with a regular one.

Another way to test for adequate corpus luteum function is for your physician to do a timed *endometrial biopsy*. This may be performed in your doctor's office and is usually a relatively painless procedure. A speculum is placed in your vagina, and a local anesthetic such as Novocaine is injected into various points of the cervix in order to block any nerve pathways that might be stimulated by a catheter or a biopsy instrument. The cervix is soft, and in itself this is not a painful injection, much less so than when the dentist makes an injection into your firm gums before filling a cavity. There are no aftereffects to having an endometrial biopsy.

You may experience some slight cramping or staining, which will not last long. But you can continue with normal activities that same day, and your period should occur at the scheduled time.

An instrument is placed onto the cervix to help steady it, while a narrow tube is pushed gently through the cervix into the uterine cavity. A piece of the lining of the uterus will then be scraped or suctioned off, by means of negative pressure using a syringe attached to the end of the instrument. The specimen is collected and sent to a gynecologic pathologist. There are also other instruments and techniques used to obtain endometrial biopsies.

The procedure must be performed late in your menstrual cycle, between days 21 to 24, the time period known as the "window of implantation," once it has been established by a pregnancy test that you are not, in fact, already pregnant. To the pathologist, your specimen will represent a certain day of the menstrual cycle, as each day causes a different appearance in the uterine lining. If there is more than a two-day discrepancy between your stated date in the cycle and the pathologist's assessment, and if there is a further discrepancy in the day your period next occurs, then we can tell whether you have a corpus luteum deficiency. Even if you are ovulating and producing progesterone, it may not be a strong enough level to support a pregnancy and the ripening egg may not be mature enough for fertilization.

Yet another way of testing for CLD is to take blood samples from your arm, at intervals beginning from the time of ovulation (about day 14), to check for levels of progesterone. If your blood levels are low, your temperature chart does not show a sustained rise, and the endometrial biopsy does not fit with your dates, then there would certainly be good evidence of corpus-luteal deficiency. Treatment will be discussed later in this chapter.

Why Doesn't the Corpus Luteum
Always Function Properly?

The formation of the corpus luteum is dependent on the secretion of hormones from the midbrain called *gonadotropins*. It has been shown that optimal pregnancy establishment and outcome occurs with conception, and therefore ovulation, between days 11 and 15 of the cycle, as the developing egg needs to be exposed to gonadotropins to enable it to undergo the best form of cell division. Psychological or stress factors that have been shown to affect the midbrain may affect gonadotropin production. Also, hormones produced by the brain work in tandem with hormones produced by the body's organs. When levels are low in one, that is reflected in the others. It is the chicken-and-egg argument: no one can pinpoint which comes first. But stress or severe emotional problems may affect your basic menstrual cycle, ability to conceive, and ability to carry a baby to term by interfering with ovulation and corpus luteum function.

Overly high secretion of another hormone called *prolactin* (the hormone mainly responsible for producing milk after delivery) may also inhibit corpus luteum function. Prolactin increase has been related to enlargement of the pituitary gland in the brain and stress. If your test shows raised levels of prolactin, you can be treated fairly easily. But often the cause of poor corpus luteum function is not found.

There are many different ways to treat a corpus luteum deficiency. Essentially the goal is to restore your body's progesterone levels. We now rely almost exclusively on natural progesterone for this treatment, the same as the hormone made by your body during pregnancy. Many women question whether taking this hormone substitute is safe in pregnancy, and whether it will lead to any birth defects. The issue has been raised because most of the currently available medications that act like progesterone are *not* natural progesterone. These synthetic hormones, known as *progestogens*, have been blamed for an increase in certain birth defects. Only natural progesterone should be used by patients trying to conceive or prevent a miscarriage. There has been no study showing any risk to your baby from the use of natural progesterone either before or during pregnancy. As usual, however, the caveat applies: no medication should ever be taken in pregnancy unless there is a specific reason and unless the risks are outweighed by the possible benefits. Natural progesterone received a bad name only because it was lumped in with synthetic progestogens.

If it is determined that you have a CLD and you are not yet pregnant, then it is a good idea to begin treatment before you conceive in order to give your next pregnancy a healthier start. Treatment can be given in a number of ways, and you should follow your doctor's advice. Right at the beginning of your menstrual cycle, you would take clomiphene, which will ensure ovulation at the correct stage of your cycle. Then you would take natural hormone progesterone suppositories, which are inserted vaginally in a dose of 50 milligrams morning and evening, from about 3 to 4 days after ovulation day (i.e., around day 18) for at least 10 days. At that point a pregnancy test would be done. If you are not pregnant, the suppositories would be discontinued. If conception does take place, then the suppositories would usually be continued well into your pregnancy, with periodic hormone-level tests conducted to ensure that your hormones levels remain adequate.

Progesterone vaginal suppositories are inconvenient in that they may drip or leak from the vagina during the course of the day. Some women complain that their vagina feels dry, and others complain of irritation. The latter side effect may be from the base chemical in which the progesterone is mixed. You could ask your pharmacist to make up the suppository in a different base.

How long into your pregnancy you continue the treatment depends on the recommendation of your doctor. Usually progesterone treatment is not necessary after about week 10—dating the pregnancy from the first day of your last period—because by then you should have adequate levels of progesterone and your doctor would have seen the developing placenta on the sonogram. Depending on your miscarriage history, however, treatment can be continued to weeks 14 to 16. Natural progesterone is also available by injection, in vaginal cream or gel form, or in tablets by mouth.

Natural progesterones given vaginally result in higher levels in the womb than oral or injected progesterone. There is yet another method of treatment in trying to increase the body's natural production of progesterone: injections of human chorionic gonadotropin, e.g. Pregnyl. Some doctors give injections of Pregnyl every few days in the second half of your menstrual cycle. But since treatment for corpus luteum deficiency is still being researched, you must rely on your doctor's advice for the best method in your case.

Can Hormone Therapy Be Enough to Prevent Miscarriage?

If you recall Ruth's story in Chapter 2, she had been put on progesterone, yet her problems were multiple. Ultimately, in her eyes, the progesterone did not seem so significant in the ensuing healthy birth. This is very often the case. You may emerge from a successful pregnancy wondering whether the hormonal treatment was necessary. But if you have had previous miscarriages, and if time is of the essence, it is wisest for your physician to treat you with the utmost caution. If hormonal therapy helps support the pregnancy through the tricky passage of the first trimester, then at least you will have come through one of the most treacherous stages safely. Progesterone problems are thought to be an important background factor in many miscarriages.

The following stories reflect related but very different situations, where doctors seem to be doing everything possible and treating anything that could have been a problem, yet the women just could not hold a pregnancy and were advised to adopt.

Martha went through three miscarriages, including the loss of a baby born alive at 20 weeks, who lived for only an hour. Finally, she suffered through a terrifying pregnancy, from which she now has her lovely 1-month-old son. Martha ran the gamut of treatments: progesterone suppositories, bed rest, antibiotics for a urinary tract infection, a cervical stitch, immune-directed treatment, and daily ingestion of one baby aspirin and vitamins. She tells her story with compassion and an intensity of feeling shared, I am sure, by many women.

"It Took Me a Month to Let Myself Wake Up to the Fact That I Had a Son!"

❦

My first miscarriage happened seven years ago, when I was 23 years old. My husband and I very much wanted this baby and were so excited by the pregnancy. It never occurred to me anything would go wrong. For the first 2 months, things were going fine. Then, at not quite 3 months, I started to spot. The doctor told me I must come in for a checkup. He did a sonogram, which showed that the fetus was not alive. It was a Friday, and I was to go in on Monday morning for a D&C.

I remember feeling badly that I had a dead baby inside of me for that whole weekend. It just didn't feel clean. Both my husband and I were very upset. We cried together but never really talked about it, until four months later when we obviously felt it was safer to talk. No tests were done at that time.

Six months later I was pregnant again. And once again, after 3 months, I lost the pregnancy. This time it happened at work. All of a sudden I was bleeding heavily. I phoned the doctor and was told to go home, stay in bed, and rest. But once back home, I was bleeding so heavily, I had to go into the bathroom where I very nearly fainted, the clots were so huge. I flushed it all down the toilet, so there was nothing left to test.

My husband and I then went for genetic counseling. I work every day in a facility for the mentally retarded, and I'm all too aware of the responsibility of bringing a mentally impaired person into the world—and just how hard such a child would be to raise. I wanted to know if this might be our problem. But the counselor said we were both genetically normal.

Then I became pregnant for the third time. Again I began spotting early on, but I took to my bed, and things were going along fairly well until week 20. We assumed all would be well this time. I remember it was December 30; during the day I'd felt crampy and gassy, but there was no staining. In the middle of the night, at two o'clock, I began having very bad cramps, which felt like gas pains. I began to suspect I was in labor.

By the time we sensed something was wrong and had set off for the hospital, I was already 5 centimeters dilated. The baby boy weighed 15 ounces and was born alive. It was a

Catholic hospital and they baptized him for me. An hour later he was dead.

This was all happening within a period of three years, and I was 26 years old. By then, I'd begun to react very strongly to friends' babies. I was jealous and resentful. I'd also begun to feel that I never wanted to get pregnant again, and I contemplated adoption.

But my husband was not too supportive of adoption. As he pointed out, no one had ever given us a reason for the miscarriages. "We haven't done all we can," he said. "We haven't been told we are *infertile.*" Still I wanted a baby so very badly. Two years had passed since we lost the baby, so I told myself I'd try one more time. A neighbor gave me the name of a doctor in the city who was the best specialist, she maintained. I remember thinking, "This is crazy—a doctor is a doctor." But finally I plucked up the courage to call, reasoning that I may as well give it one last try.

My husband and I went to see him together. I remember sitting there before this doctor, wondering what he could know that the others didn't. First, he gave me a complete examination and ran all sorts of tests. I'd also brought my files from the other doctors. Then he said, "Why did you wait so long after the last miscarriage?" I told him I'd been looking into adoption. He used those magic words: "There's no reason why you can't have a perfectly normal child."

He ran numerous hormone tests and thyroid tests. Eventually, after an extensive battery of tests, we went for immune testing. The testing revealed that I was not producing something in my blood to block antibodies that were rejecting the pregnancies. I was given immune-directed treatment. I have to admit that we were fearful because we might be fooling with nature; the procedure was so new and difficult to understand.

For the first 1½ to 2 months, the next pregnancy went well. There was no spotting. But then it started again, about 8 weeks into the pregnancy. I was losing blood. The doctor did blood tests and immediately noticed a problem with my hormone levels. I started on progesterone suppositories. Each week, I went to a laboratory to have blood tests, checking that the hormone levels remained adequate. From the beginning, I was told to take one baby aspirin a day, to increase the blood supply going to the placenta. And I was put on antibiotics for a urinary infection. So, while pregnant, I was taking progesterone suppositories, erythromycin [the antibiotic], baby aspirin, vitamins, and I had received immune treatment. I was worried the whole way through!

Apart from visits to the doctor and to the laboratory, I was on *complete* bed rest. To make matters worse, I was physically sick, vomiting night and day, and I couldn't eat anything. At the 4th month, the doctor put a stitch in my cervix. But still I woke up one night with cramps and found to my horror that there was blood all over the sheets. I phoned the doctor in a panic, crying that I'd lost the baby. He told me to relax and come to see him in the morning. By this time I was resigned to yet another loss. I'd been so sick, and through so much, it was almost a relief to think the pregnancy was over.

The doctor gave me a sonogram. The heartbeat was there; even I could see the heartbeat! In truth, I felt a little exhausted that it wasn't all over. This was becoming quite a struggle. But the doctor told me the pregnancy looked very healthy.

Two weeks later, I returned for another sonogram. The doctor had seen an empty sac and he now explained that I had been carrying twins and had lost one of them.

After 5 months, my sickness and vomiting finally stopped, and I began to feel like a normal pregnant person, except for the constant fear every time I went to the bathroom where I would check myself. I continued having regular ultrasound scans. The doctor took out the cervical stitch a week before my due date, in case I went into labor. In the end, a week overdue, I wasn't having contractions, and he induced me. I went into the hospital at 9:00 A.M., and at 12:58 P.M. I delivered my son. He was perfectly normal.

He's so big already, maybe it was from all those drugs I was taking. I'd love another baby but I'm not sure about putting myself through all that again. I'm 30 years old and I realize how lucky I was to have started young.

It wasn't until I saw the baby coming out of me, I thought, Oh, my God, this is it! At first I kept rather cool and unemotional. Then I began to cry. It took about a month until I let myself wake up to the fact that we had a son. My husband still can't believe he is a father. Every night we go in and look at our son asleep, in wonderment.

⚘

"I'd Reached the Point of Giving Up. The IVF Doctor Recommended Either an Egg Donor or Adoption"

Evelyn says her problems with pregnancy must have been due to her advanced age. She was 38 when they started trying to have a baby. Now at 41, a very charming, attractive lawyer, she looks much younger than her age. Seven months pregnant, she exudes a contented look of happy pregnancy. She really wants to warn other women in their late thirties not to wait too long if they want to have a baby. There really is not much time once you are near-ing 40, especially if things begin to go wrong.

❦

The very first time we tried to get pregnant, I conceived in a couple of months. It was mid-August and I was about 10½ weeks. Coming home by subway, I started bleeding. When I saw that it was bright red blood, I knew that was bad. My doctor at the time advised me to rest and keep my feet raised. But in the morning, I saw the mucus plug come out. I went for a sonogram and there was no heartbeat. The doctor talked to me about having a D&C, but I didn't want to risk the surgical procedure, so I waited a week. That was terrible. It didn't come out fully, so I had to have the curettage in the end.

While we were on vacation in Italy, 9/11 happened. I took it very badly as my commute had been through the World Trade Center. I just didn't want to try getting pregnant again for a while. The next spring, we had another go, and similarly within a couple of months I was pregnant. This time, my ob/gyn saw me earlier and I had more regular sonograms. At 5 weeks, we heard the heartbeat and I was feeling great. At 12 weeks, I went for a regular sonogram and there was no heart-beat. This time I accepted having the D&C. About 18 months had now gone by and time was running out for me, or so I felt.

My sister has a friend who'd gone through 11 miscarriages. I made an appointment for three months ahead with the doc-tor she had used. I just was not prepared to take any further risks. He did all the blood work and one of the tests revealed very high natural killer cells and also the blood-clotting factor. He put me on Lovenox, a blood thinner [heparin], baby aspirin, progesterone, and prednisone. I was also taking Clomid. I became pregnant immediately and went in for blood tests every day. But my hormone levels were not increasing properly. This time it was a blighted ovum and it just came out naturally.

Because of my history and age (by now I was 40), he suggested I try IVF and also pre-implantation genetic testing (PGD), as that way they can choose better embryos. It took several months to be accepted onto the program I wanted. That spring, I began injections of fertility drugs and taking baby aspirin. The daily sonograms show how many eggs you've produced. It's like a chicken hatchery! I produced eight, four on each side. When they retrieved them, they took just four and from those two actually fertilized. It was last year, on Mother's Day, that they implanted them and said that they were the best quality. I was feeling very positive.

It didn't work. There was no pregnancy. My husband and I were so upset that we stopped trying for a few months. Then you slip out of the program cycle and have to wait to get back in. Once I was ready to start again, my blood tests began to show a raised level of the hormone estradiol, which meant I couldn't proceed. The next month, my FSH level was too high. Nothing seemed to be going right. I was devastated and have to admit I began to give up. The IVF doctor had been quite negative about my chances of succeeding. High hormone levels lead to difficulties getting pregnant and also a higher incidence of miscarriage. He suggested I consider either an egg donor or adoption.

Someone I knew recommended I try acupuncture. We de-

cided to drop out of the IVF program and se
pregnant again on our own. We'd done i
reached my limits with all the testing and ir
did go for an acupuncture session the night I
lating.

Then I found out I was pregnant the natural way. I called
the doctor, who immediately ran blood tests and continued
doing so every couple of days, to ensure the hormone levels
were rising adequately. It was all very scary as I was used to
getting negative results from these tests. I also had a sonogram
every two weeks. At 5 weeks there was a heartbeat. He traced
the tissue from the previous two miscarriages and that seemed
to show that I have the factor which causes blood clotting. I
began taking baby aspirin and folic acid. But I just didn't want
to take all that other medication, such as the prednisone, this
time. If it was meant to be, it would happen, was my feeling
by now.

I had the nuchal translucency ultrasound and blood tests,
rather than the amniocentesis with its own risks of miscarriage. The risk levels were low for the pregnancy. I've since
had a couple of high-resolution sonograms. But, apart from
that, I've had quite a normal pregnancy. Now I'm at 34 weeks
and I'm beginning to relax, because after 7 months the fetus is
viable. That's why I tell my friends now, that if they're saying
"maybe not yet, not quite the right time," they should think
again. Especially if you're nearing 40. You never know how
long it might take.

❦

Shortly after this interview, Evelyn gave birth to a healthy
daughter.

Other Hormonal Causes of Miscarriage

Abnormalities

lities of thyroid function, including an underactive thy-
cause a miscarriage. Thyroid function is checked by a
st and, if it is abnormal, treatment is given to keep the
thyroid-stimulating hormone (TSH) in the normal

Prolactin

ctin is a hormone secreted from the midbrain. A raised pro-
in level can also interfere with the formation of the corpus lu-
eum and lead to pregnancy loss. The level of this hormone must
be measured and treated if it is high.

Polycystic Ovarian Syndrome (PCOS)

This common hormonal disorder occurs in 5 to 10 percent of
young women. It is associated with an increased production of
male hormones (androgens) such as testosterone. This causes irregular ovulation and irregular menstrual periods, resulting in
difficulty in getting pregnant. Women with PCOS can suffer
weight problems, acne, and increased hair growth, although none
of these symptoms may occur.

PCOS is diagnosed by a combination of ultrasound of the
ovaries and blood tests to measure various hormone levels. A fea-
ture of this condition is that it is often associated with insulin
hormone resistance, which increases the risk of first-trimester
miscarriage and the development of gestational (pregnancy-
induced) diabetes. If insulin resistance is found, the patient can
be treated with an oral antidiabetic drug such as metformin (Glu-

cophage). This will decrease the miscarriage risk and lower the chances of the development of gestational diabetes.

Diabetes
Uncontrolled diabetes may lead to miscarriage and pregnancy loss. The condition should be controlled before a woman becomes pregnant. In pregnancy, your doctor will work closely with your diabetic specialist and you should have a completely normal pregnancy.

The Magic Dance of Life

Why is it so easy for some women to conceive and give birth to healthy babies, and so hard for others? Why is it that some women are fertile, whereas you and your partner, who so very much want a baby, seem doomed to pain and loss?

These major questions, no doubt, plague you almost every day of your life if you have miscarried more than once. There is not, as you already know, a simple answer. But at this point I think it would be sensible to introduce a description of the basic female reproductive anatomy, so that we are all comfortable with the terms and concepts under discussion.

The Organs of Reproduction

Although most women today probably feel they know as much as they'll ever need to about their female sexual or reproductive parts, let me explain how they are classified in medical terminology. The vagina is the passageway to the internal organs; the ovaries offer a place for the storage and production of eggs; the fallopian tubes provide a site for fertilization and the passageway for transportation of the fertilized egg or blastocyst; the uterus is the site for implantation of the developing fetus.

The External Genitalia

The external genitalia include the vulva, the area between your upper thighs, which includes the mons pubis, labia majora, labia minora, clitoris, hymen, urethral opening, and various glandular structures. (See Figure 7.)

The mons pubis is a fat-filled cushion, covered by curly pubic hair, which is in a triangular-shaped pattern in the female. The labia majora are two rounded folds of fat, covered in tissue, similar to the scrotum in the male. In young girls, the labia majora lie close together, whereas in women who have had children the labia may gape. Following puberty the labia are covered with hair, which extends onto the inner thighs.

The labia minora, reddish in color, vary greatly in size. After

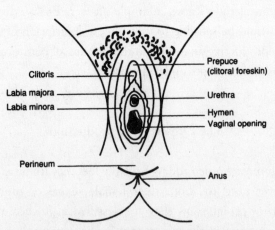

Figure 7. Above is a drawing showing the normal
anatomy of the vulva.

childbirth they can project out. Their thin folds of tissue enfold nerve endings, and their muscles can make them erectile.

The clitoris is the equivalent to the male penis, a small erectile body that rarely exceeds 2 centimeters in length even in a state of erection. The clitoris is extremely sensitive to touch, being one of the principal female erogenous zones.

The urethra is the opening to the bladder. Close by, just under it, is the vaginal opening, which varies in size and shape in different women. A tubular or hollow muscular structure between the bladder and rectum, the vagina is the major female organ of copulation. It can vary considerably in length, though it is usually about 10 centimeters long. In childbirth, however, it will distend markedly. The lower portion of the cervix, which is the entrance to the uterus, or womb, projects into the top of the vagina.

The Internal Genitalia

Figure 8 shows the internal genitalia. The portion of the cervix visible from the vagina has an opening in its center known as the external os. Before childbirth it is small and oval, but it changes in shape after the birth of a first child. The other end of the cervix, which opens into the lower portion of the uterus, has an opening known as the internal os. The cervix is only a few centimeters in length.

The cervix is composed mainly of smooth muscle, collagen fibers, and blood vessels. During pregnancy the collagen tissue becomes flexible so that it will separate and soften. Normally the percentage of muscle content is fairly low, around 10 percent. However, in a woman with an incompetent cervix, the proportion of muscle in the makeup of the cervix is appreciably lower. The glands in the canal, or passage, in the cervix secrete a mucus that provides a protective plug during pregnancy. When it is dis-

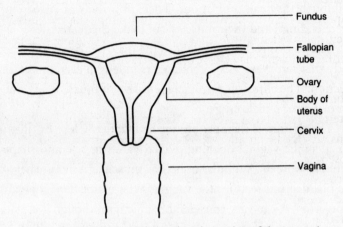

Figure 8. This drawing shows the relationship of the internal
genital organs.

charged at the onset of labor, it is called the "show." The isthmus
between the body of the uterus and the cervix stretches during
late pregnancy and labor, forming the lower segment or lower part
of the uterus through which C-sections are done if needed.

The uterus is a muscular organ, the shape of which has often
been likened to an inverted pear. It has a cavity lined with tissue,
known as the endometrium, which in turn nourishes the fetus in
pregnancy under the influence of progesterone. This endometrium
is a thick, pink velvetlike membrane, varying in depth from 0.5 to 5
millimeters, lined with blood vessels. The endometrial cells undergo
many changes that, as we saw earlier in this chapter, can be recognized at each stage by the pathologist during the menstrual cycle.

The fallopian tubes come out of the cornua, or angles, at each
side at the top of the uterus. They vary in length from 6 to 10
centimeters and will shrink markedly after menopause. They also
vary in diameter from 2 to 3 millimeters to 5 to 8 millimeters.
Like the endometrium, the tubes are lined with a mucus membrane. This lining is composed of only a single layer of cells, and

it also undergoes changes throughout the cycle, changes that are important for a woman's fertility. For example, if the lining has been damaged, the tube may not be able to support fertilization satisfactorily and may be a cause of sterility.

Each fallopian tube is divided into four parts: the part of the tube that runs through the wall of the uterus and then up into the external part of the tube (the interstitial portion); the part that runs next to the uterine wall (the isthmical portion); and the place close to the ovary where fertilization takes place (the ampullary portion). The final part, at the end of the tube, extends in finger-like structures called fimbria to the surface of the ovary, ready to surround the egg like the tentacles of an octopus, as it is slowly expelled from the surface of the ovary at the time of ovulation. The egg, once released, is transported along the tube by hairlike cells helped by contractions of the walls of the tube.

The ovaries are almond-shaped organs that develop and produce eggs. They also secrete their own share of hormones. The ovaries vary in size from 2.5 to 5 centimeters in length and shrink after menopause. They are located in the upper part of the pelvis, on its back wall, lying between two large blood vessels and behind the fallopian tubes.

The Endometrium and Hormonal Change

There are three changes to the endometrium (lining of the uterine cavity) each month that are very important in the reproductive chain:

1. Menstrual phase
2. Follicular or proliferative phase
3. Luteal or secretory phase

Following a menstrual period (menstrual phase), the endometrium is thin, since the blood-vessel lining has been completely shed. It gradually builds up and becomes thicker (follicular or proliferative phase), until it reaches the stage when it is thick and nourishing (secretory or luteal phase) again. These changes are brought about by the timed release of hormones during the menstrual cycle.

At the time of menstruation, for example, the midbrain produces gonadotropin-releasing hormones that travel down to the pituitary gland lower in the brain. In turn, gonadotropins are then released; at first, the main hormone is follicle-stimulating hormone (FSH). FSH travels through the bloodstream to the ovary, where it causes an egg (or *follicle*) to ripen. The very act of ripening causes the egg to produce the hormone estrogen, which in turn triggers the endometrial lining to begin developing once again (proliferative phase).

At midcycle, around day 14, another gonadotropin is secreted by the pituitary gland in the brain called luteinizing hormone (LH), and this causes the egg to leave the ovary (ovulation). The period from the onset of menstruation to ovulation lasts about 14 days, but in reality it may vary between 8 and 20 days. The second part of the cycle is more exact: from ovulation it takes exactly 14 days before the onset of your next period, unless you become pregnant. So, you always ovulate 14 days *before* your next period, not necessarily 14 days from the start of your last period.

The moment of release of the egg is not a sudden act, as many women believe. In fact, it takes place quite slowly over a period of two to three minutes. The expulsion of the egg may also be accompanied by a little spillage of fluid from the now empty structure (the follicle). If the fluid spills into the pelvic cavity, it may be accompanied by a little pain or cramping. This is the mittelschmerz—a midcycle sensation of lower abdominal pain—

lasting only a few hours. Some mucus or blood may also be released into the vagina (ovulation cascade). Both are not only common, but good signs of ovulation.

The egg is then picked up by a fallopian tube. The pituitary
gland continues to secrete the gonadotropin LH, which also
causes the follicle that expelled the egg to produce progesterone
(as well as estrogen). The follicle is now called the corpus luteum.
LH is secreted for 14 days, at which time the corpus luteum
(which with conception would persist to support the early pregnancy) degenerates and a new cycle starts over with the onset of
the menstrual phase. (See Figure 9.)

The production of progesterone during the luteal phase is

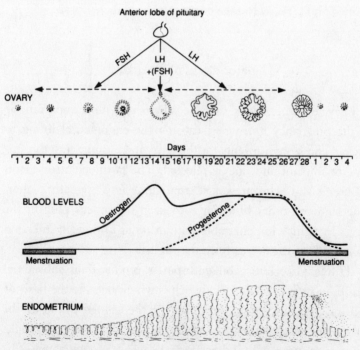

Figure 9. This diagram shows the hormonal control (FSH, LH)
of the ovary and endometrial lining of the uterus.

very important in maintaining a pregnancy. When the egg is fertilized, LH will continue to be secreted, and the corpus luteum will not degenerate but continue to produce progesterone. It is progesterone that makes the endometrium secretory, building nutrients for the early fertilized egg.

When a pregnancy occurs, the message to the corpus luteum not to die after 14 days, and to the endometrial membrane to continue its secretions, comes from the pregnancy hormone, human chorionic gonadotropin or HCG, which has in itself been produced by the fertilized egg. So, it is the fertilized egg that gives the signal to keep producing progesterone, to keep itself alive, and well nourished. HCG stops the corpus luteum from degenerating for at least the first 8 to 9 weeks, until the placenta has developed and is ready to take over nourishing the embryo.

The Hormones of Pregnancy

As I have explained, progesterone is by far the most important of all the pregnancy hormones, causing the endometrial lining to thicken and store nutrients for the fetus and encouraging the embryo to implant and not be rejected. The hormone also sedates the uterus and helps prevent it from going into premature labor. Progesterone's other function is to keep the mucus plug in the cervix in a thick impenetrable state in order to prevent infection from entering the uterus from the vagina.

Human chorionic gonadotropin is produced in substantial quantities during pregnancy, which is why it became the basis of the first pregnancy tests. Produced by the cellular lining of the early fertilized egg, it helps keep the corpus luteum alive. Its highest concentration is found at 10 to 12 weeks of pregnancy. The level then drops throughout the ensuing months, although it remains raised throughout pregnancy. If you receive a blood test showing your HCG level is stable or dropping toward the end of the first trimester, that is probably quite normal.

Estrogen and many other hormones are also produced but are not given for the treatment of recurrent miscarriages.

The Uterus, Fallopian Tubes, and Ovaries

If there are any defects in these three major organs, problems with reproduction can arise. Incredibly they were developed, in *you*, at a very early embryonic stage. For example, the uterus and fallopian tubes in a female embryo develop in the 5th week after fertilization, at which point the embryo is only about 10 to 11 millimeters long. The uterus begins as two halves. After these two sections fuse, the developing uterus begins to form a cavity that is finally completed by the time the fetus is 12 weeks old. The vaginal opening, however, is not complete until the 6th month of pregnancy.

During this early stage of embryonic development, the two halves of the uterus may fail to fuse together properly or fuse only partially, giving rise to anatomical problems.

Similarly, problems may arise in utero with the ovaries and the production of eggs. The cells that are going to form eggs appear in the female fetus approximately 3 weeks after conception! At 2 months, the female embryo has about 600,000 eggs. By 5 months, the embryo is storing nearly 7 million eggs. By the time the baby is born, that number will have dropped to 2 million, and, by puberty, it will have dropped even further to around 400,000.

Women need only a few hundred eggs for the purposes of reproduction, as only one egg tends to be released each cycle. But this huge store of eggs slowly declines during the woman's reproductive life. By the time a woman is 35, the number of eggs has dwindled from 400,000 at puberty, to 35,000.

As far as is known, women do not form new eggs after birth, whereas men constantly manufacture fresh sperm on a daily basis. Many millions of sperm may be ejaculated in a single act of intercourse, and sperm begin forming again almost immediately.

The Menstrual Cycle and Human Ovulation

A regular menstrual cycle throughout the reproductive years has great significance. Each month the drama of life is being reenacted: maturation of an egg, ovulation, potential fertilization, and implantation. The whole system is very complex and not that well understood. There are many academic groups and societies, such as the Society for the Investigation of Early Pregnancy (SIEP), that are in the forefront of investigating how pregnancy occurs and how problems can best be treated.

However, we do know about the predictable changes of hormone production and the cyclic production of eggs at approximately one-month intervals. It is most unusual for a woman to be permanently anovulatory (unable to produce an egg and unlikely to menstruate).

So the major significance of regular periods is that the whole cycle is normal; it probably means that you are ovulating and have normal levels of the sex hormones. If you are ovulating, we assume your production of gonadotropin-releasing hormone, follicle-stimulating hormone, luteinizing hormone from the brain, and progesterone and estrogen from the ovary is appropriate.

The ovulatory cycle and the endometrial cycle (changes in the endometrial lining of the uterine cavity) are intimately related, and they are reflected in hormone activity.

One of the great mysteries of the human reproductive cycle is why so few of the many thousands of eggs are ever selected to ripen, and further, why certain eggs ripen and others do not.

When ovulation takes place, often more than one egg or follicle starts to ripen, but usually only one or two follicles make their way to the surface of the ovary, at which point the ovarian wall becomes thinner. The follicle picks a site where the rupture will occur. The mature human ovum is barely visible to the naked eye. The corpus luteum forms in the ovary at the site of the ruptured follicle. Its name literally means "yellow body" because it is a bright gold color. It measures about 1 to 3 centimeters in diameter and can easily be seen by the naked eye.

The time of ovulation in the menstrual cycle is very important because fertilization must take place within hours of ovulation. To get a better idea as to when you should try to conceive, start assessing your own cycle by recording the onset of your next period, which will be exactly 14 days after you last ovulated.

As many as 25 percent of women are aware of their ovulation. They may have some symptoms of the mittelschmerz, which I mentioned earlier. Or, they might be aware of a higher basal temperature, which is measured by a special thermometer. Ovulation, in fact, occurs just *before* the shift in your temperature, which is caused by the action of progesterone produced after ovulation. To keep a temperature chart you should get a special thermometer and graph recording page from your doctor or pharmacist. You must take your temperature orally (or rectally) for three minutes before getting out of bed in the morning. The widely spaced graph paper will display the temperature shift that occurs after ovulation.

. There are all kinds of do-it-yourself ovulation predictor tests to measure the rise in LH, which triggers ovulation. Such commercial tests, together with temperature charts, are among the best methods of judging when ovulation occurs, and thus when conception could take place if you have intercourse.

How the Embryo and Fetus Develop Throughout a Pregnancy

The moment of conception is the beginning of the dramatic and exciting development of new human life. The potential fate of this meeting of sperm and egg in the outer part of the fallopian tube may be foretold within the first few hours, or days, following fertilization.

The cells then fuse and immediately start to divide; by day 4 there is a mass of cells called the *blastocyst*. This develops little fingerlike structures, known as chorionic villi, which are necessary for the embedding of the developing embryo. After day 7, the embryo reaches the uterus. The villi start burrowing into the lining of the uterus, and the embryo receives a new source of nutrition by opening into the mother's blood vessels. The outer surfaces of the villi are covered in a special substance that keeps blood flowing around it and doesn't allow it to clot.

The First Trimester

The mass of cells begins to form into an embryo and an amniotic sac. As the embryo develops, a cord goes out to the yet-to-be-formed placenta. Amniotic fluid is put into production, and the amniotic and chorionic membranes appear.

Normal pregnancy dates from the first day of your last period. But, to be more accurate, I use a method that refers to the moment of conception (day 14 of that cycle). So, when I say "2 weeks after conception," that would be the same as week 4 of normal pregnancy dating, or the time of your first missed period.

By 2 weeks after conception (i.e., week 4) the pregnancy is large enough to be seen by the naked eye. The ovary still contains the tiny corpus luteum, which is supporting the conception.

By 3 weeks after conception, the embryo is 2 millimeters long. Its major organs, such as the spine, nervous system, head, and trunk, are just starting to take shape.

By 4 weeks after conception, the head is formed, and the chest, abdomen, brain, and spinal cord are complete. Limb buds begin to appear, and by the end of this week the heart is formed and circulation begins.

By 5 weeks after conception, the limbs develop. The baby's own blood cells start circulating throughout its body. The intestines are growing, but they are not yet in their proper place. The embryo is now 1.3 centimeters (about ½ inch) long.

By 6 weeks the heart starts beating strongly. All the major internal organs, including the lungs, are formed. Growth of the eyes and ears is now taking place. The embryo is 2.2 centimeters (nearly 1 inch) long. This is the very worst time for the mother to be in contact with German measles (rubella), as the fetal eyes and ears would be directly involved. An ultrasound scan should now be able to show the fetal heart pulsing, and the viability of the pregnancy can be assessed.

By the end of 7 weeks, the embryo is about 3 centimeters long (just over 1¼ inches) and weighs 2 grams (less than ⅛ ounce). Although the baby can now move, you will not feel it for some time yet.

By 8 weeks, the umbilical cord is formed, but there is still not a placenta in working order. The embryo is 4.5 centimeters (1¾ inches) long and weighs 5 grams (less than ¼ ounce).

By 9 weeks after conception (week 11), the embryo is recognizable as a human being. Its eyes are completely formed, and it is now be classified as a fetus. It is about as long as your little finger, 5.5 centimeters (2¼ inches), and weighs 10 grams (⅓ ounce).

All the major organs are formed within these 9 weeks after conception, the period of *organogenesis*. From this time on, therefore, the fetus is not subject to major congenital catastrophes, although it may be affected by environmental hazards or premature delivery.

By 10 weeks the face is completely formed, and the external genital organs are forming. The baby is 6.5 centimeters (2½ inches) long and weighs 18 grams (nearly ⅔ ounce).

By 11 weeks from conception (week 13), the sex of the baby may possibly be seen on an ultrasound scan (if it is a boy, at least). The fetus is about 7.5 centimeters (3 inches) long and weighs 30 grams (about 1 ounce).

The 12th week after conception marks the end of the first trimester, when all the organs are formed but the baby is still immature. The fetus, as we have seen, could not live independently outside of the uterus.

The uterus is now so enlarged that it begins to protrude out of the pelvis, and your doctor should be able to palpate it (feel the uterus with his or her hands) abdominally. The uterus also now contains about 100 milliliters (less than 1 cup) of amniotic fluid.

The object of the pregnancy from this point on is to help the baby further mature so that it can survive outside the womb.

The Second Trimester

By 13 weeks from conception (week 15), bodily changes become evident in the fetus. The neck has lengthened and its head no longer rests on its chest. The abdominal wall closes, concealing the intestines, which until then have been on the outside.

By 14 weeks the baby's joints start moving; fingernails and toenails have grown. A fine downy hair called *lanugo* covers the entire body. The baby is also covered with a greasy substance called *vernix*, which protects its skin from the watery amniotic environment. The fetus is now 16 centimeters (6¼ inches) long and weighs 35 grams (1¼ ounces).

From the 15th to the 18th week, the fetus grows rapidly in both its length and weight. It has hair on its head and because of increased muscle development it will begin to make some very active movements that the mother can feel. There is still a relatively large amount of amniotic fluid in which the baby is swimming. The fetus is now 25.5 centimeters (10 inches) long, and its weight begins to jump to around 340 grams (nearly 12 ounces).

By 22 weeks after conception, the baby is about 35.5 centimeters (14 inches) long and weighs about 570 grams (1¼ pounds).

By 26 weeks, the baby's head is only slightly larger in proportion to its body size, so it takes on the appearance of a more normal baby. It should be about 37 centimeters (14½ inches) long and weigh around 900 grams (nearly 2 pounds).

From the 26th week, the fetus can be regarded as viable—capable of independent life in the outside world, although highly dependent on neonatal care. Birth from this time on is called premature. Legally the baby must be registered, and if it dies, the baby will require burial. Neonatal care gives an almost 70 percent chance of survival at this stage, but there are many, many risks along the way in the next few weeks.

The Third Trimester

At the beginning of this trimester, the baby is still covered with a greasy vernix, and its lungs are not mature, which of course offers the main problem for the neonatologists.

By 30 weeks after conception, the baby is perfectly formed.

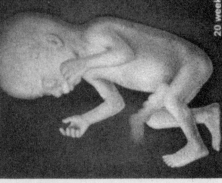

6 weeks

- Embryo almost 1 inch in length
- 1/30 of an ounce in weight
- Inception of eyes, ears, and nose
- Evolution of digestive system
- Backbone appears
- Budding arms, elbows, and fingers
- Budding legs, knees, and toes
- Formation of face and features

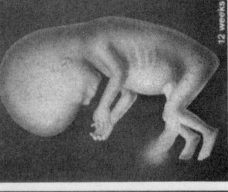

12 weeks

- Fetus almost 3 inches in length
- 1/2 to 1 ounce in weight
- Hands, fingers, and nails now distinct
- Feet, toes, and nails now distinct
- Evidence of baby teeth outgrowth
- Most bones have commenced development
- Kidneys begin to secrete urine
- External sex organs become more definite

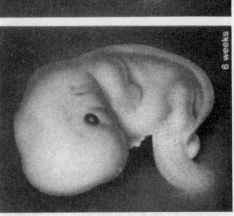

20 weeks

- Fetus almost 10 inches in length
- 8 to 12 ounces in weight
- External sex organs now fully defined
- Well-formed eyes, ears, nose, and mouth
- Bronchial tube branching becomes evident
- Heart sounds perceptible with stethoscope
- "Cheesy" protective covering on skin
- Hair on head, "down" on body
- Mother may feel baby's movement (quickening)

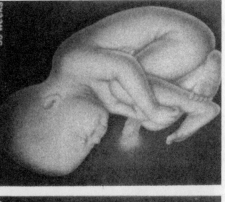

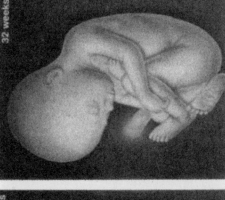

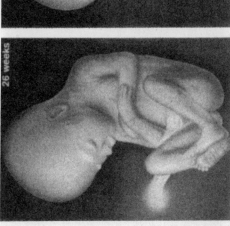

26 weeks

- Fetus almost 14 inches in length
- 1½ pounds in weight
- Skin appears red and wrinkled
- "Cheesy" film covering still on skin
- Eyelashes well defined
- Eyebrows well defined
- Nostrils now open

32 weeks

- Fetus almost 16 inches in length
- 4 pounds in weight
- Internal organs more completely developed
- Body filling out
- Eyelids now open
- Bones fully evolved but still soft and flexible

38 weeks

- Fetus almost 19 inches in length
- 6 pounds in weight
- Hair on head now thicker and longer
- "Down" disappearing on body
- Fingernails reach fingertips
- Skin loses wrinkled appearance; now smooth
- Slate-colored eyes usually change color after birth

Figure 10. Stages of development of a human baby.

The head is in proportion to the body, and the baby has a good chance of survival if born. The baby is about 40.5 centimeters (16 inches) long and weighs about 1.6 kilograms (3½ pounds).

At 36 weeks, the baby is considered fully mature. Its organs are not only formed but are working normally. The baby can survive if born now, or if induced or delivered by C-section, and it should not have a problem breathing because by now its lungs are mature. The baby is about 46 centimeters (18 inches) long and weighs about 2.5 kilograms (5½ pounds).

By 38 weeks after conception (the classic 40 weeks of full-term birth), the baby is ready to be born. The fine body hair called lanugo has disappeared, and the baby has early head hair. Its eyes will be slate blue (all babies are born with blue eyes, though the color often changes within weeks after birth). The nails are properly grown. It will have put on a lot of body fat in the past month to give a chubby, healthy appearance at birth.

At full-term a baby may be as long as 50 centimeters (nearly 20 inches) and will weigh an average of 3.5 kilograms (7½ pounds).

Is There a Link Between Infertility and Miscarriage?

Many women who have noticed that they go through periods of infertility wonder if they run a greater than average risk of miscarrying. It might be terribly worrisome for a couple who is struggling with problems of conception to imagine having to face the tragedy of a miscarriage. But you should not blind yourselves to one very basic fact: the same cause may be triggering both effects.

Increasingly, medical research is coming to view the process of reproduction as a continuum: problems with fertility, miscarriage, and premature delivery are viewed as links in the same fragmented chain.

About 15 to 20 percent of clinical pregnancies, those that are identified by a positive pregnancy test and a missed period, miscarry. We now know an equal number of pregnancies fail even before they are apparent. They are called *chemical pregnancies* and can be diagnosed by doing highly sensitive tests in the second half of the menstrual cycle, measuring levels of the pregnancy hormone HCG. It is now believed that some cases of unexplained infertility are due to earlier recurrent pregnancy losses (chemical pregnancies). The couple is successful in conceiving but miscarries very early. Have you ever felt or suspected you were pregnant, and then your period has come, which was somewhat heavier than usual? Many women mention this. Poor implantation at days 21–24 of the menstrual cycle sets the stage for miscarriage or other late-pregnancy problems such as growth retardation and pre-eclampsia.

So if you have previously been treated for infertility problems, you should be followed very closely by your doctor once a pregnancy is achieved. Your HCG levels will be monitored, as well as your progesterone levels. You may be treated with progesterone suppositories in the early weeks of pregnancy, as an inadequate corpus luteum may be the root cause.

Bear in mind, however, that the statistics for rates of miscarriage among such a high-risk group may appear artificially high because of the close scrutiny given these pregnancies. If you miscarry after receiving a very early positive pregnancy test, the loss will be recorded, whereas another woman might not even have known she was pregnant.

One in six Americans of childbearing age is now thought to be infertile. That accounts for 10 million men and women. The numbers of infertile couples are growing, too. One in four women age 35 and over are said to be infertile. Even more worrisome: about 5 percent of women in their early twenties, a figure that has increased in the past 20 years, are now having problems conceiving. Couples are thought to have an infertility problem if they have tried for a pregnancy for a year or they are in their midthirties and have tried unsuccessfully for six to eight months. With such statistics in mind, you won't be surprised by women's and men's quickly mounting sense of despair at their problems.

Michelle's story demonstrates why no one should ever give up, and also the link between apparent infertility and miscarriages. She's a hardworking psychologist with a busy practice who now has two sons, aged 3½ and 1½. Her path to motherhood did not progress at all as she'd imagined when she began trying to get pregnant at nearly 30.

"I'd Had Five Attempts at IVF. Two Ended in Miscarriages, and the Rest Failed to Get Me Pregnant"

❦

In all those years I was trying to get pregnant, I went to loads of doctors, including all the well-known ones. I had IVF, but kept on miscarrying. I'd already had five attempts at IVF. Two ended in miscarriages; the rest failed to get me pregnant. I also had six inseminations that failed.

Finally, I was introduced to a doctor who tested me for immune problems. When he saw my records he could see the problems very clearly. I had stage 5 endometriosis, also PCOS [polycystic ovarian syndrome], and there was an immunological problem. I live an hour away from his office, but I would have traveled 10 hours if necessary. I came across him from attending an infertility conference and listening to his lecture. My husband and I were both tested, and finally, for the last pregnancy, I was given IVIG every three weeks during the first trimester. I was also on heparin twice a day throughout the pregnancy, and baby aspirin. The first baby was born without problems.

But I had different problems with my second child. I was given IVIG and went through IVF to conceive. I became very sick and had to be hospitalized, as I was suffering chest problems and trouble with breathing. I was put on a massive dose of steroids (prednisone) throughout the pregnancy. No one ever really knew what was causing my problems or whether the medication would affect the baby. There were a lot of serious ethical issues involved. Thank God everything was okay. In the end, I was induced and given more steroids. Then the baby himself got sick and had to be put on steroids. He wouldn't sleep or eat and I had round-the-clock nursing. But my kids, both of them, are absolutely fine now and very healthy. They are just pure miracles!

I didn't want to continue IVF without any explanation of why it kept failing. You're paying all that money, but no immune tests were given to see if I might in fact miscarry. The reason given for this lack of testing is that there is no exact correlation, no hard evidence. They also point to the fact that IVIG is a blood product and therefore could possibly lead to future problems.

There is no question that IVIG is a controversial medication. Although some doctors adamantly refuse to use it, women are so desperate they will go to any lengths to find the treatment. It's already in use for autoimmune diseases. Also, the fact that insurance companies won't approve its usage makes it very expensive.

My doctor is the one person who has really changed my life. I can't ever express my gratitude. He's given me my children. When I was so sick and lying there in the hospital, not knowing what was going on, he came to visit and sat there holding my hand. He really gives people hope—even when you have lost all hope. And I should know, as I've been to every doctor under the sun!

6

Can Ordinary Infections or
a Virus Cause a Miscarriage?

If you catch a bad cold, suffer from influenza ("flu") during pregnancy, or run a fever, it can be very frightening. If you then go on to miscarry, you may think the virus was the cause of your loss, even though this is probably not so. In fact, we are trying to learn more about the role played by infections in recurrent miscarriages. Some infections may be hidden and not lead to symptoms. The good news is that many of these asymptomatic infections are treatable. Some have also been pinpointed as likely causes of infertility. If an infection that can cause fertility problems is diagnosed, you may be advised to take a course of antibiotics before becoming pregnant, and then remain on this antibiotic treatment for at least some part of the pregnancy.

Most bacterial, viral, and fungal infections can cause sporadic pregnancy loss. The organisms most likely to do this are listeria, toxoplasma, and viruses such as herpes, measles, and those causing flu. However, when we come to the question of the causes of recurrent pregnancy loss, the evidence is uncertain and is still the subject of research. New knowledge and skills in treating these infections are yet other factors in today's management of recurrent miscarriages. There is much research under way about the link between infections and subsequent infertility, miscarriage, and other obstetric problems such as premature labor.

Infections may act in the first trimester of pregnancy. They may be present in the woman's genital tract or travel into the womb on the sperm, causing an inflammatory response, which can then damage the embryo or its implantation in the womb.

Later in the pregnancy, after 12 weeks, infections can be carried through the bloodstream or from the vagina through an incompetent cervix. If the mother's waters are broken or leaking, infections may also reach the fetus and the pregnancy may be lost as a consequence. Any infections associated with a very high fever can cause pregnancy loss or lead to premature labor.

The exact relationship between a specific infection and a miscarriage is not always easy to prove. The infection, for example, that emerges in a test performed after a miscarriage might have occurred only following the death of this fetus. The vagina always contains certain organisms, and, in principle, any organism *could* cause a miscarriage if it gained access to the uterine cavity. But rest assured: organisms do not usually reach the uterus in later pregnancy as the increased acidity of the vagina and the mucus plug in the cervix block their path. Nonetheless, if your miscarriage was not obviously caused by other major problems, some of which have been discussed in previous chapters, then it is important that you and your partner be tested for infections. Your partner's sperm and seminal fluid must be cultured for infections.

Infections and Diseases That May Cause Miscarriage

Many bacteria have been cited as causes of miscarriages. In theory, they travel through the mother's bloodstream and across the placenta to the fetus, but most bacteria are too large to cross the placental barrier. Still, much needs to be learned about the association between bacterial infection and miscarriage. Below is a discussion of some infections that have been implicated in miscarriage. Some are well documented, while others are newer discoveries.

Mycoplasma Hominis and Ureaplasma Urealyticum

These organisms have been linked with recurrent miscarriage. They lead to a low-grade subclinical infection, that is, an infection that does not cause any symptoms in the mother. You would show no signs of abnormality, as mycoplasma hominis and ureaplasma urealyticum are also found in normal fertile women. Mycoplasma hominis is a cross between a bacteria and a virus and lives in either the female or male genital tracts. The organism acts by causing chronic infection in the endometrium, or uterine lining. If you noticed a fever following a prior miscarriage, this may be a sign of infection.

Mycoplasma hominis was only identified as a cause of recurrent miscarriage in 1978, when studies identified a special kind of mycoplasma, called the T-strain, that was found in many women who had experienced recurrent miscarriages.

To test for the organism, we take a vaginal culture from the mother and a sterile semen sample from the father. Both mother and father have to be tested. Between pregnancies, mycoplasma hominis and ureaplasma urealyticum can also be diagnosed by taking a biopsy of the inside of the uterine cavity (endometrial biopsy). If either is identified, before you try for another pregnancy you and your partner would each be given a course of antibiotics, usually doxycycline (a form of tetracycline), for two weeks. If it is not discovered until you are already pregnant, treatment is available using an antibiotic that is safe in pregnancy.

Syphillis

Although now rare, this disease used to be known as the Great Aborter. Its incidence is now on the rise again and it certainly does cause miscarriages. It can affect the fetus at any time during pregnancy, but especially in the beginning, at conception.

Bacterial Vaginosis

This organism is quite common and can cause a creamy vaginal discharge with a fishy odor. It has been associated with second-trimester miscarriages and is a cause of premature labor, so it must be treated if discovered in a pregnant woman.

Toxoplasmosis

Another infection that is likely to carry no symptoms, toxoplasmosis has been identified as a possible cause of sporadic or recurrent miscarriages. It is important to be able to make the diagnosis through either blood tests or endometrial biopsy. If the parasite is found, you would have to be treated for the infection.

Toxoplasmosis is a parasitic infection transmitted by household pets and is known to lead to miscarriage, birth defects, premature labor, and stillbirth. Having said that, and alarming every cat owner in the nation, let me reassure you that its occurrence is very rare, about 1 in 8000 pregnant women. There is no cause for alarm or need to move the cat out of the house during your pregnancy. *Just do not handle cat litter if you are pregnant.* Either relegate the task to your partner or, if you have no other choice, use rubber gloves to change the litter box. This is especially important if you do not have immunity to the organism. Some of us, however, are already immune to toxoplasmosis, having lived around household pets all our lives.

Exposure to cat feces is not the only way to acquire toxoplasmosis. One can also become infected by eating raw meat such as steak tartare or raw fish such as sushi. Many women in Europe and Japan have become immune to toxoplasmosis as a result of their exposure to raw meat and fish. But it is wiser that you avoid these foods in pregnancy. You will often be tested for immunity to toxoplasmosis as part of the prenatal blood-test package.

Group B Streptococcus

This organism is often cultured for in late pregnancy. If group B steptococcus is present, the mother will be treated with an antibiotic on going into labor so that the baby doesn't become infected as it passes through the vagina during delivery. While the organism is associated with newborn problems, it is not associated with early pregnancy loss.

Chlamydia

One of the most common sexually transmitted organisms today is chlamydia. It is especially common among the young and sexually active and has been associated with impairment of fertility, so testing for chlamydia is now almost routine. Carriers of chlamydia are usually unaware of the infection because it causes no symptoms.

Present in the genital and urinary tracts of men and women, the organism does not invade the placenta or uterus, so we are not altogether sure of its role in causing a miscarriage, but it has been isolated from tissue following a miscarriage. To test for it, your doctor takes a swab from the cervix, much like a Pap smear. If chlamydia is diagnosed, both members of the couple are treated with a course of antibiotics.

Listeria

This bacterium is associated with miscarriage. A team of microbiologists from Leeds, England, showed that at least one-quarter of test samples of precooked chilled meats from supermarkets was contaminated with listeria, which has been shown to harm unborn, or even newborn, babies. Listeria may be present because shorter heating times are used for prepared foods. Thorough cooking of meats will destroy the bacteria. Listeria has also been found in cheeses made from nonpasteurized milk. There is a case on record of a pregnancy loss at 21 weeks from infected goat's milk cheese.

Pregnant women should be aware of the danger of eating partially cooked foods, including chicken, turkey, beef, and spare ribs. They should also avoid soft cheeses or those made from unpasteurized milk. While listeria can cause a miscarriage, it is a self-limiting disease and does not cause recurrent pregnancy loss. Women can be tested via an endometrial biopsy or cervical swab.

Monilia

Monilia, a yeast infection, is a very common cause of vaginitis, which occurs with increased frequency in pregnancy because of an elevated sugar content in the vaginal cells and the high acidity of the vagina itself. Monilia has been associated with miscarriage, but only when an intrauterine device has been in place. The IUD may itself be the cause of miscarrying the pregnancy. If monilia is present in pregnancy, it should be treated, because it causes discomfort and may also infect the baby as it passes through the vagina. It can also cause an episiotomy to heal poorly. Safe treatment with nystatin is possible in pregnancy.

Malaria

Malaria can cause a miscarriage, probably because of the associated high fever or circulatory disturbance in the placenta. But this is not usually a cause for concern unless you have been traveling in parts of the world where malaria is endemic. It would be advisable to avoid such areas in early pregnancy.

Viruses

As is the case with bacteria, the exact roles of viruses in miscarriages is unknown. There are several difficulties in assessing the role of viruses. First, it is difficult to isolate a virus from miscarried tissue. Second, viral disease is common both in and out of pregnancy. Even the common cold has been implicated in sporadic miscarriages. Yet there are certain viruses that are known to be dangerous in pregnancy. It is not known how they get to the pregnancy, but they probably spread through the bloodstream.

Rubella (German Measles)

The rubella virus crosses the placenta and infects both the placenta and fetal tissue, causing either congenital abnormalities or a spontaneous miscarriage. We do not know how often miscarriages are caused by rubella, as most reports focus on the abnormalities found at birth if the pregnancy continues.

Genital Herpes

Genital herpes may cause a miscarriage if you have the *initial* attack in early pregnancy—during the first 20 weeks. It is believed that the virus may cross the placenta and infect the embryo or fetus; or it may act by interfering with the correct recognition of the father's protein in the embryo by disrupting the antigen G (see Chapter 8). Usually, the first attack of herpes is more severe than recurring attacks and is accompanied by a high fever. It is not known whether the fever or the herpes virus actually causes the miscarriage.

If you have already had an attack of herpes and become pregnant, the recurring attacks are not believed to cause a miscarriage or any fetal abnormalities. So do not be concerned if you or your husband have a history of herpes. A recurring attack will only be significant in pregnancy if it causes a lesion, or ulcer, on the cervix, vagina, or labia that is still present when you go into labor. In that case, you would require delivery by C-section to avoid the baby's coming into contact with the virus in the ulcer. Antiviral drugs are not safe to use during pregnancy.

Other Viruses

HIV (human immunodeficiency virus; also known as the AIDS virus) does not cause miscarriage, but it can be associated with general maternal illness, which may be a cause. Cytomegalovirus, commonly found in AIDS patients, was once thought to be a cause of miscarriages, although no known link has yet been discovered. Mumps, measles, hepatitis A and B, parvovirus B19 (Fifth disease), and coxsackievirus may also be linked to miscarriage.

Can You Be Vaccinated During Pregnancy?

Is it safe for the fetus? is the question asked by so many women who require vaccination during pregnancy. This is one of those complex issues that needs to be talked through seriously with your doctor; the pros and cons will have to be weighed by you and your partner before making a decision. As a general rule, it is thought that the fetus is more endangered by *live vaccines,* for example, those against rabies, yellow fever, polio, smallpox, mumps, measles, rubella, and chickenpox (varicella). Vaccination with dead or inactivated vaccines, such as those for whooping cough, typhoid, cholera, influenza, and polio are safe in pregnancy.

Rubella Vaccine

While rubella is preventable by vaccination before you are pregnant, you cannot be vaccinated against rubella once pregnant. Although the virus in the vaccination is weak, it is nevertheless alive and could damage the fetus. You should have a blood test done before you get pregnant to see if you need to be immunized against the disease.

If you are not immune, you should not get pregnant for the next three months after vaccination. If you are already pregnant, you should be vaccinated immediately after delivery, before you leave the hospital, to protect you and the fetus in any future pregnancy. It is safe to breastfeed after the vaccination.

Flu Vaccine

Though common, influenza is an epidemic disease and, as the vaccine is safe, it is recommended that all pregnant women be vaccinated during flu season. Influenza can be more severe in pregnancy.

Tetanus Toxoid Vaccine

Given as a booster against a possible tetanus risk, this vaccine is safe in pregnancy.

Infections Associated with Certain Procedures

Insertion of the Cervical Stitch (Shirodkar)

The later a stitch is inserted into the cervix, say, after 18 weeks, the greater the chance of infection occurring. This may cause the membranes to become infected, thus possibly causing the fetus to be affected or the membranes to rupture. We are not sure why there is greater protection if the stitch is placed earlier. Antibiotics may be given following the procedure as a precaution. This is also one reason why the stitch should be removed about two weeks before you expect to go into labor, as it will give your body time to destroy any cervical infection associated with the stitch and will prevent the uterus from becoming infected after delivery.

IUD in Place

If your pregnancy is diagnosed while you have an intrauterine device still in place, infection may be a significant problem, as the IUD acts as a foreign body in the uterus, promoting infection. There is a greater risk of infection if the strings of the device are protruding into the vagina, as they may act as a track for infection to follow into the uterus. The doctor usually removes the device if the strings are visible.

Intercourse

Apart from the prostaglandins in semen, which have been mentioned as a potential cause of difficulties if you have previously miscarried, there is another reason to be cautious about intercourse if miscarriage is a potential problem: bacteria can be carried on the sperm. If you are in the second trimester, and your cervix is short or already slightly open, bacteria may enter the uterus. This could lead to infection and rupture of the membranes or increased uterine contractions. These risks do not apply in a normal pregnancy, where intercourse is not forbidden at any stage.

The human female is the only mammal that mates during pregnancy, and bacteria in the vagina do represent a challenge. In late pregnancy beta streptococcus is now cultured for routinely, with a swab taken from the vagina. However, it is not a cause of miscarriage and is only treated in labor to prevent infection of the baby as it passes through the birth canal.

If vaginal intercourse is prohibited, anal intercourse should be avoided.

Rely on your doctor's advice regarding intercourse in high-risk pregnancy situations. The use of a condom may be advised in some circumstances.

7

✿

Diseases and Disorders in the
Mother or the Father

Maternal Diseases

Diabetes Mellitus
Some people strongly believe that diabetes is associated with an increased risk of miscarriage. However, this has not been conclusively demonstrated. Just as with systemic lupus erythematosus (SLE), if the illness is controlled, the miscarriage rate doesn't rise.

There is no increase in miscarriages in *gestational* diabetics, that is, in patients who have diabetes only when pregnant (which has resulted from pregnancy hormones interfering with the action of insulin). This is screened for routinely at 28 weeks with a one-hour measurement of your blood sugar level after being given a sweet drink. If the results are not normal, then you have a glucose-tolerance test: glucose is given as a drink and the blood sugar level is tested for up to three hours after the drink. But studies have shown increased miscarriage rates in *frank uncontrolled* diabetes, known as type 1 or insulin-dependent diabetes. Even then, however, miscarriage is avoidable, and there should be no increase in miscarriage rate if a patient's diabetes is controlled.

A glucose-tolerance test is therefore not necessary as part of a routine workup in recurrent miscarriage. Sometimes a random glucose measurement is taken of the blood, however, just to be certain. If glucose is elevated, further testing is done.

Thyroid Disorders

Although there is still no firm evidence that thyroid disorders are associated with recurrent miscarriage, historically women with an underactive thyroid have been seen to be at greater risk. Although many research studies have tried to prove a definite link, so far without success, thyroid testing is done routinely in patients who undergo recurrent miscarriages. A blood sample is sent to the laboratory to test for thyroid function, in particular, for levels of thyroid-stimulating hormone (TSH). Because both hypothyroidism (underactive thyroid) and hyperthyroidism (overactive thyroid) have been linked to increased miscarriage rates, the test is important. Thyroid replacement medication for an underactive thyroid is safe during pregnancy. If you have hypothyroidism, your blood will also be tested for antithyroid antibodies, as they may be causing your thyroid to underact. These antibodies may cause a miscarriage and can be treated if present.

Endometriosis

This is a common disorder and a cause of infertility in women of reproductive age. Some studies also suggest that it may cause miscarriages, though the exact basis for this is not understood. But it is now known that endometriosis is an autoimmune disease and may be associated with autoantibodies, such as antiphospholipid antibodies (APAs), which are a known cause of miscarriage. The miscarriage rate is thought to be lower in women whose endometriosis is treated, either medically or surgically.

Systemic Lupus Erythematosis

Systemic lupus erythematosis is an autoimmune disturbance in which the person forms antibodies against his or her *own* tissues. It is a much more common disorder in women than in men, and unfortunately it affects women particularly in their childbearing years. SLE is one illness that has been associated with an increased rate of miscarriage in part because there is an increased incidence of antibodies. We are not sure why this kind of miscarriage occurs, but antibodies are the probable cause. You should be tested for SLE if your doctor is running tests for the causes of miscarriage; a blood sample is tested for one of the antinuclear antibodies (ANA).

Fortunately, medical treatment using steroids, such as prednisone, is effective in keeping SLE under control and has allowed women with this disease to carry pregnancies to term.

Usually women with SLE are already aware of the condition, and their doctors treat such pregnancies with due care and caution. Without treatment the miscarriage rate would be as high as 30 percent. Usually the loss occurs between the 2nd and 3rd month of the pregnancy in untreated cases.

Recently, it has been theorized that the ANA group of antibodies may be present well before the onset of clinical lupus. Could it be that recurrent miscarriage is a marker for the possible future development of lupus or another autoimmune disorder? This is not currently proven, but has been suggested in recent medical literature.

Heart Disease

If you were born with certain types of congenital heart disease, you may be more likely to miscarry, because the fetus may not receive adequate oxygen from your circulation. This does *not* apply to women with heart murmurs or mitral valve prolapse (MVP), which is a benign condition increasingly diagnosed in otherwise healthy young women.

Migraine

Migraines, while common in pregnancy, are not a cause of miscarriage, but ergotamine compounds may not be used to treat the condition in pregnancy.

Coagulation Disorders

These have been discussed previously under thrombophilias (factors that promote clotting). Abnormalities in blood platelets have been associated with pregnancy loss (von Willebrand disease), though not necessarily so. If you have a family history of this type of condition or any other bleeding problems, you should be tested and treated before you conceive.

Blood Groups

Human blood contains proteins of different types or groups. Two major groups are the ABO and the Rh groups. In pregnancy, if not before, you will be aware of your own group. Studies about the role of ABO blood group incompatibility between the parents, as a possible cause of either infertility or recurrent miscarriage, have been inconclusive.

However, the Rh blood group is important, because if the mother is Rh negative and the father is Rh positive, there is a chance that the mother may make antibodies to the baby's blood. This is known as Rh disease. Fortunately, Rh disease is preventable using shots of Rhogam (anti-D) routinely at 28 weeks of pregnancy; if any bleeding occurs; and after birth. If the mother develops Rh disease, the antibodies formed in her blood can cause drastic problems in pregnancy, ranging from miscarriage to stillbirth.

There is a rare blood group system, called the P system. If the father has the P system in his blood, the mother may form antibodies and this may cause miscarriage. Fortunately it is very rare and is not routinely tested for.

Liver Disease

This is not a cause of recurrent miscarriage, though a rare condition called Wilson's disease, a disturbance of copper metabolism, has been associated with pregnancy loss. It can be tested by measuring a substance called caeruloplasmin in the mother's blood and can be successfully treated.

Other Diseases

Other chronic maternal illnesses, such as pulmonary (lung) and renal (kidney) disease are also causes of pregnancy loss. In all probability, this is due to a disturbance in the blood flow to the embryo and the placenta.

Blood Flow to the Womb

Very recently scientific studies have suggested that testing for adequate blood flow through the mother's arteries into her womb is important in treating infertile patients and in early pregnancy. It is thought that a decrease in the blood flow may cause a miscarriage or interfere with later fetal development. This is tested for by ultrasound and may help to identify a cause of recurrent early pregnancy loss. It is a new area of investigation and not at present part of routine testing. However, it may provide information about the possible causes of some disorders of fertility and early pregnancy. It will also indicate the best methods of treatment for those conditions.

The Endometrial Function Test

Earlier I have mentioned that many cases of unexplained infertility may in fact be undiagnosed recurrent chemical pregnancies. When the fertilized egg fails to implant in the uterine wall, this will lead to loss of pregnancy before you have even achieved a positive pregnancy test.

A group of Yale University researchers has developed a new method of testing specimens (biopsies) of the lining of the womb. Besides looking at uterine lining structure, they can now analyze the lining to see if it contains substances called markers, which may affect the embryo's implanting. These various markers are numerous and are still being researched. But the tests may well be worth doing before IVF is undertaken, as they might reveal the cause of previously unexplained infertility.

Paternal Disorders

The husband or partner cannot be left out when it comes to preventing miscarriage. Male factors contributing to pregnancy loss include chromosomal abnormalities in the father's sperm. There is now evidence that men may have problems in the protein composition of the sperm. This can be investigated through a sperm DNA integrity test (SDI) and should be performed on husbands or partners of women who have suffered recurrent miscarriage (especially if the miscarriage tissue chromosomes were male) or unexplained infertility. This test is only done at special laboratories.

Infections in the seminal fluid may be carried on the sperm into the uterus and might lead to early pregnancy loss. The seminal fluid should therefore be cultured, in a sterile semen sample, and sent to a laboratory for testing. In particular, mycoplasma hominis and ureaplasma must be tested for.

Alcoholism in the male is commonly seen as playing a part in pregnancy loss. Whether this is due to the extra stress experienced by the mother or to actual damage to the sperm by the alcohol is still not known.

High numbers of abnormally shaped sperm may be a factor in recurrent miscarriage. It has also been questioned whether too many sperm (over 250 million per milliliter), known as polyspermy, may be a cause of miscarriage.

Immunologic problems involving seminal fluid have been reported, such as the presence of increased immune cells, but the exact role this plays in miscarriage is not yet certain.

While more reasons for the father's contribution to recurrent pregnancy loss are being discovered, there is still little conclusive evidence. Nonetheless, it is important to investigate both partners rather than just focus on the mother.

Placental Disorders

We used to think until a few years ago that abnormal shapes or attachments of the placenta caused pregnancy loss. However, now it is believed that many pregnancy problems, including chemical pregnancies, early or late pregnancy loss, poor growth of the fetus, premature labor, pre-eclampsia, and stillbirth, all may be due to the initial poor implantation of the embryo in the mother's womb and faulty connection to her blood supply. This may be caused by an imbalance in the immune response. If the balance is upset, the inflammatory cytokines (T-helper type 1, or TH1) overwhelm the protective cytokines (TH2 group), and the implantation is dislocated, with the resultant pregnancy problems listed previously. Such an imbalance may result from poor immune signaling between mother and embryo at the time of implantation.

The Histopathology of Early Pregnancy Loss

Until recently, tissue removed by D&C following a miscarriage was sent for routine testing, but its value was largely disregarded. Essentially, it was used to confirm that the patient had been pregnant and that it was not a tubal (ectopic) pregnancy.

However, this tissue is the vital junction between the mother and the embryo or fetus, and a careful analysis can give valuable information as to what caused the pregnancy to die. This critical review is done by a group of perinatal pathologists. They will be looking, for example, to see whether the pregnancy failure was caused by blood clotting interfering with the mother-to-baby blood flow; by an infection; or by immune damage. It may even be possible to tell if there was a chromosome problem, which is very useful if genetic testing was not requested at the time the tissue was obtained.

Similar reviews can be done, too, on any earlier miscarriages you may have had, by requesting the tissue slides from the hospital or pathology laboratory where it was sent (slides are kept for 20 years by laboratories). All of this evidence can help support the results of other blood tests and can guide the doctor's future treatment plans.

Stress and Anxiety

The human being has a very powerful and well-controlled nervous system, and it is known that our nerves, or stress and anxiety, can affect our immunologic and hormonal systems. Even so much more needs to be known about the effects of stress, and it is now being studied much more carefully.

Because it occurs in early pregnancy, we used to believe that spontaneous miscarriage was an event of less serious emotional consequence compared with other forms of bereavement. But now it is widely acknowledged that women who experience miscarriages, and particularly those who undergo recurrent miscarriages, may undergo intense and serious grief reactions that can deeply affect their quality of life.

Relieving stress and anxiety is important in pregnancy as, apart from anything else, it will make the difficult period of undergoing tests, and subsequent pregnancy, a more comfortable experience. There really are beneficial effects to psychological support for women who have undergone several miscarriages. Tender loving care (TLC) and, of course, good medical care certainly contribute to a higher success rate in pregnancy.

It is thought, however, that stress may contribute to infertility and pregnancy loss by disrupting the finely tuned hormonal pathways and immunologic responses of the reproductive system. This has already been shown to be the case in animal studies by Petra Arck and her colleagues in Berlin, where immune balances were upset in the uterine lining of mice when they miscarried following stress induced by exposure to sound waves.

The quality of care you receive is extremely important. Reassurance, constant support, medical treatment if necessary, and frequent ultrasound scans to see the fetal heartbeat all help the mother to see that her pregnancy is healthy and progressing well. I believe that a firm, but informed, positive attitude can be tremendously helpful.

If you are very preoccupied with and upset about your miscarriages, it might be advisable to consult a psychologist, social worker, or counselor trained in pregnancy loss. You may want to attend such sessions with your husband or partner, as, even if he appears to be adopting the stiff-upper-lip approach, he may be masking deeper emotions. Relaxation techniques such as acupuncture, yoga, and massage can also be helpful. Although one of the softer aspects of science, the role of stress and anxiety is an intriguing one that needs to be solved with further research.

8

ℱ

Immunological Causes of Miscarriages: Is There a Mismatch Between You, Your Partner, and the Baby?

When you are happily pregnant, nurturing the unborn in your swelling abdomen, you would never think to reject it as something foreign to you; nothing could be further from your thoughts. But your body may in fact be reacting to foreign tissue in what, outside of pregnancy, would be considered a very normal manner.

The Immunologic Paradox of Pregnancy

Immunological research is one of the most exciting new areas of science today. Essentially, immunology is the study of the body's internal response to invaders: foreign substances it doesn't recognize and sets out to destroy in order to protect you. We are accustomed to hearing about this in terms of skin or organ transplants, in which the race against time is to provide sufficient immuno-suppressant drugs to stop the body from rejecting the foreign tissue. Just think, then, how unusual is the state of pregnancy, in which 50 percent of the embryo is of foreign (to the mother) tissue, having been contributed by the father. Not only does the mother's body accept this foreign tissue, but it actively nurtures it for 40 weeks!

Although this new area of science is still somewhat controversial, couples who experience unexplained infertility, recurrent miscarriages, pregnancy loss, or repeated IVF failures should be screened for immunological problems.

This fascinating high-tech field of immunology within the realm of miscarriage research has already helped many thousands of women and their partners. The classic case offered immunologic testing is the woman who repeatedly miscarries early for no obvious reason. It is now believed that immunologic causes account for a large percentage of previously unexplained recurrent miscarriages. This means that many women may be eligible for this type of help. The treatments are still considered controversial and experimental because, just as in IVF treatments and other areas of medicine, not every mechanism of how something works is understood. Nevertheless, studies show good success rates for immunologic treatment and the immunologic reasons for miscarriage are being seen as more and more important. For women who have given up hope of carrying a pregnancy safely to term, this is very encouraging news. Immunologic investigation and treatment are certainly breakthroughs. Many couples, who would otherwise have been childless, now have one or more children as a result of this new approach.

What Are the Immunological Problems
of Pregnancy?

In fact, it is less surprising that some pregnant women's bodies reject their fetuses than that any fetus makes it through to full-term birth. Why? Because the processes of conception, fertilization, and embryological development go against one of the basic tenets of nature. The body, as transplant surgeons well know, rejects anything it does not recognize as its own. The embryo is only 50 percent its mother's tissue; the other half, which comes from the father, is foreign tissue to her body, known in immunology as a semi-allograft.

In the very early days following conception, the *trophoblast*, the bundle of fetal cells of the developing embryo and placenta, actually comes in contact with the mother's tissue and her blood as it attaches to the uterine wall.

A pregnant woman normally reacts to the embryo, but while making an immune response; it is of a protective type, which allows the embryo a privileged position and helps it to grow. These protective, growth-promoting special substances, called cytokines, produced by immune cells in the wall of the uterus called T cells, allow the pregnancy to survive. (See Figure 11.)

No one is certain how this occurs. One theory is that the mother's immune cells recognize a protein in the father's half of the embryo, sometimes called antigen G, and are triggered to make the appropriate protective response. There also seem to be substances in the man's semen that block the mother's T cells from recognizing the embryo as foreign. There are probably also other immune mechanisms that we have yet to discover that allow the embryo to implant and survive.

We don't yet fully understand why there is a breakdown in these mechanisms for some couples. It could be due to a fault in the interaction of the basic genetic makeup of the mother and father. Some believe that a woman who becomes pregnant has naturally been exposed to her partner's cells through intercourse; that these tissue proteins called antigens (proteins that trigger an antibody response) are carried in the semen; and that this exposure helps her body to produce the protective rather than the destructive inflammatory cytokines. Some women's bodies just may not recognize their partners' tissue correctly.

Doctors used to think that in pregnancy the mother's immune system was suppressed. In fact, it is the immune system's *failure* to recognize this tissue as *foreign enough* that prevents the correct type of response from being made—not, as you might imagine, a wildly aggressive immune system attacking all foreign tissue at will. It is now believed that certain men and women are genetically too similar for this recognition to occur. As a result, the woman adopts her husband's antigens as her own and does not produce the protective response. Miscarriage or unexplained infertility may then occur.

There is no way of knowing beforehand who will be affected, though it does lend credibility to the biblical injunction against marrying a first cousin or a very close relative. The problem is asymptomatic—there is no high temperature or nausea. And how much you love your partner bears not the slightest relevance.

From the moment the fertilized egg starts to implant, between days 21 and 24 of the cycle, this very early embryo, or trophoblast, must attach to the mother's womb to receive its blood supply. As half of the embryo is foreign to the mother, it is vital that there be correct signaling between the mother's immune cells in the lining of the uterus (which are there to protect her from infection) and the embryo. If the signaling is correct, the pregnancy grows and develops to become a healthy birth. The same process will also determine the quality of health for the newborn child.

There is now compelling evidence that in addition to the protective immune response described above, there are *other* immune factors in the mother's blood that can lead to reproductive or pregnancy problems. Their impact can come at different stages of the reproductive cycle, making sense of unexplained infertility, recurrent miscarriages, poor growth of the baby during pregnancy, pre-eclampsia, stillbirth, or repeated failure of IVF. These immune factors include antiphospholipid antibodies, antithyroid antibodies, and, most recently discovered, elevated levels of the natural killer cells. The good news is that there are tests to investigate all these conditions in special laboratories.

Other Immune Tests and Their Treatments

Natural Killer Cells

Your doctor will evaluate you for possible immune problems in a very new way by measuring some of your immune cell levels, including your natural killer cells, in a process called *immunophenotyping*. We all have natural killer cells in our bodies. They're important as protectors, killing off tumor cells and virally infected cells. If these are too plentiful, they can cause a miscarriage by attacking the embryo. If levels of NK cells are elevated, the condition can often be treated successfully using the drug intravenous immune globulin (IVIG). Although still controversial and regarded as experimental, there is growing evidence for the successful outcome of pregnancy in women who suffer recurrent miscarriages and those who repeatedly fail IVF by using IVIG treatment.

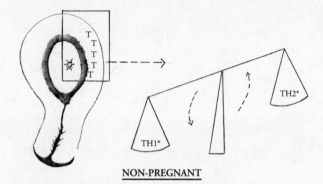

<u>NON-PREGNANT</u>

Presence of germ in uterus causes a destructive immune response by
mother's T cells.
TH1* Destructive Inflammatory Immune Response (TH1)
TH2* Protective Immune Response (TH2)
T = T cells in uterine wall
☀= germ

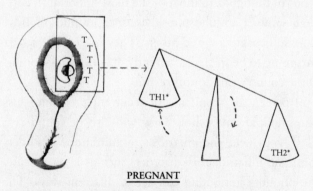

<u>PREGNANT</u>

In pregnancy, immune signals between embryo and mother favors a shift in
balance from destructive to protective response.
TH1* Destructive Inflammatory Immune Response (TH1)
TH2* Protective Immune Response (TH2)
T = T cells in uterine wall
◑ = embryo
◀ = father's half of the embryo

Figure 11. Immune response and the embryo.

Thrombophilias

Another immunologic problem is the presence of thrombophilias, clotting factors that interfere with the blood supply to the pregnancy. You may have been born with them (hereditary) or developed them later in life (acquired), especially if you have had miscarriages.

Hereditary thrombophilias occur in women with strong family histories of high blood pressure, strokes, or heart attacks. Thrombophilias can be identified by a panel of tests done by various commercial laboratories. New components are constantly being discovered. The most important ones for our purposes are protein S, protein C, Leyden V mutation, MTHFR mutation, homocysteine, and prothombin 20210A.

Acquired thrombophilias, also called antiphospholipid antibodies or APAs, are being actively researched, and new types are still being added to the list. They include anticardiolipin (the most well known, though certainly not the most important); antiphosphoethanolamine; antiphosphotidylserine; antiphosphotidyl glycerol; lupus anticoagulant, and others. They must all be tested for if you are going to be treated. Currently only certain laboratories around the country can do this testing.

About 50 percent of women with recurrent pregnancy loss have antiphospholipid antibodies. They will also be found at a raised level if you have endometriosis, autoimmune disorders such as lupus, and inflammatory disorders such as Lyme disease. The antiphospholipid antibodies can act in different ways. The most usual is to cut off the blood supply (by clotting) to the developing embryo or fetus and cause the heartbeat to disappear, usually resulting in a missed abortion. They may "unglue" the cells of the growing embryo and cause very early pregnancy loss, before the level of HCG has had time to rise very high before falling. They may also damage the implantation of the embryo, as it tries to attach to the uterus around days 21 to 24 of your cycle. This is a very important cause of unexplained infertility, as pregnancy tests are never positive in such cases.

Women with thrombophilias are treated with heparin and baby aspirin. Their pregnancies are also treated as high-risk as there is an increased risk of high blood pressure (pre-eclampsia) and placental separation (abruption). The condition may also interfere with the transfer of nutrition (glucose) across the placenta, resulting in growth retardation of the baby.

Antinuclear Antibodies

These antibodies react against the cell nucleus, the controlling center of a cell. They are present in autoimmune diseases such as lupus and rheumatoid arthritis. The antibodies can also be found in women on certain medications or those with vascular conditions. These antibodies can cause miscarriages and IVF failure, as they attack the embryo or placenta. Until these were discovered, women with this problem usually were not able to have children. The good news now is that all this has changed and, with treatment, these women can now bear healthy babies. Treatment is usually given in the form of steroids such as prednisone or dexamethasone by mouth.

Antithyroid Antibodies

You may have antibodies to your thyroid, even if you have normal thyroid function. They may increase your risk of recurrent pregnancy loss and they are also associated with IVF failure. Depending on your particular history, they can be treated with prednisone, dexamethasone, or IVIG.

DQ-α Testing

This test is a special type of tissue typing done on both the mother's and father's blood to see if they share the gene DQ-α, as that can result in repeated early miscarriages. It may also cause harmful autoantibodies such as antiphospholipid antibodies to be produced in early pregnancy. The treatment may be IVIG, depending on your particular history of pregnancy loss.

LAD-Lymphocyte Antibody Detection Testing

The test assesses whether the mother's body recognizes her husband's contribution to the embryo correctly. As has been described earlier, the father's portion of the embryo contains a protein, unique to him, often called antigen G. The theory is that the immune cells (T cells) in the mother's uterine lining must recognize the father's antigen G correctly and produce the necessary protective response to support the embryo. If her tissues are too genetically similar to his, she may not make the protective response, and, as a result, the pregnancy may fail to implant or miscarry later. This may also happen if the embryo fails to produce enough antigen G.

Blood is drawn from both mother and father for this test. Treatment currently is with IVIG. This condition used to be treated by immunizing or vaccinating the mother with her husband's white blood cells, which also contain his antigen G protein; however, that method of treatment has been discontinued.

Tumor Necrosis Factor

Tumor necrosis factor (TNF-α) is the inflammatory cytokine produced by the body's NK cells to destroy cancer cells and virally infected cells. High levels in the uterine lining (as obtained by endometrial biopsy) mean that the NK cells may destroy the embryo by stopping implantation and causing a miscarriage. This condition is treated with IVIG. Also, significantly raised levels of TNF-α can be measured directly in a blood sample. Increased NK cell toxicity has been associated with miscarriages, fetal loss, and unexplained infertility.

Embryotoxic Factors

T cells make cytokines. Some promote growth (TH2 variety) and some stop or kill growth (TH1 variety). This test looks for cytokines that kill embryos (TH1 type producing TNF-α). Embryotoxic factors are found in up to 6 percent of women with recurrent miscarriages and have been reported in women with endometriosis-associated infertility. IVIG can be a successful treatment for this condition.

Ratio of TH1 to TH2 Cytokine

This new blood test measures the balance between the inflammatory (TH1) cytokines and the pregnancy-protective (TH2) cytokines. In pregnancy the balance should shift toward the TH2 cytokines. If not, the condition is treated with IVIG.

Treatments for Immunologic Disorders

When investigating unexplained infertility, pregnancy loss, or failed IVF, often more than one abnormality is found on testing; for example, raised NK cells and raised APAs. Therefore, treatments may need to be combined to maximize the chance of a successful pregnancy.

Prednisone

Autoantibodies such as ANAs, APAs, and antithyroid can be treated with prednisone. Prednisone, a steroid that lowers antibody levels and encourages suppression of the immune responses, may be given early in the conception cycle. It is usually not continued beyond week 10 of pregnancy. In high doses, given for long periods, it may cause high blood pressure, diabetes, and bone thinning, so it is carefully monitored. However, because of the low dose used in pregnancy, these side effects are rare. If given later in pregnancy, prednisone may cause gestational diabetes and premature rupture of the membranes.

Aspirin

Baby aspirin (81milligrams) is usually combined with heparin in treating women with antiphospholipid antibodies and recurrent pregnancy losses or if they have infertility of immune causes. It improves blood flow, acting differently from heparin by affecting blood platelets. Low-dose aspirin has minimal side effects, if any. It must not be used if you are allergic to aspirin. It does not affect the embryo or fetus adversely and is usually continued until the 36th week of pregnancy.

Heparin

Most experts recognize blood clotting as a proven, treatable cause of recurrent pregnancy loss. In such cases, heparin injections are the treatment of choice. These may be given twice daily. The newer, low-molecular-weight heparins are longer-acting and usually need only be given once daily. They also have fewer side effects, but they are more expensive.

Your doctor or a nurse will teach you how to inject heparin subcutaneously, usually in the skin below the belly button (as it might leave a slight stain). As heparin can thin the bones, calcium supplements (1500 milligrams daily) are given by mouth. Your blood will also be drawn each month to check that the heparin dose is correct and that it is not affecting blood clotting adversely, or dropping the blood platelet levels.

Heparin and aspirin are usually given until about 36 weeks of pregnancy. They are stopped before labor, as you may not be able to have an epidural if you go into labor while taking either medication. The low dose of heparin used in pregnancy should not cause excess bleeding, though bruising at the injection site is common.

Heparin does not cross the placenta and is safe in pregnancy. It must be started soon after ovulation, before you miss your period and are diagnosed as pregnant, to be maximally effective.

Intravenous Immune Globulin: Indications and Administration

Intravenous immune globulin (IVIG) acts by lowering the level of harmful or inflammatory antibodies or cytokines produced by Natural Killer cells. It also blocks all autoantibodies, such as antiphospholipid and antithyroid antibodies. It is usually recommended for treatment of women whose bodies have been shown not to recognize their husband's contribution to the embryo correctly (as shown in a LAD test), those with increased NK cells, a positive embryotoxic factor, unexplained recurrent miscarriages, or repeated IVF failures. Many such women who might previously have given up hope are now producing healthy babies after treatment.

IVIG has been used by doctors for over 28 years to treat autoimmune diseases such as multiple sclerosis, but it is new in the treatment of miscarriage and IVF failure. This is an "off-label" use for the drug—a new use for an already approved drug. Unfortunately, IVIG is very expensive, almost $2500 per dose, and some insurance companies will not cover it for this off-label use. The product is made from many human blood donors. Great care is taken to kill any viruses or other infections. Not only are the blood donors screened, but the product is heated twice and washed with a detergent that kills all viruses. Unless some unknown disease is discovered in the future, the product can be considered safe. No transmission of HIV (AIDS) has ever been reported in the United States or in the UK in all the years of its usage. You must be careful to request a detergent-washed product.

IVIG therapy for treatment of pregnancy problems such as recurrent miscarriage is considered experimental and it is not yet an approved drug for use in pregnancy, although limited published studies have shown it to be beneficial. Informed consent must be obtained, and you will have to be fully advised about IVIG and its side effects. You will have a blood test (total IgA) as 1 woman in 800 who fail this test cannot receive the drug safely for fear of a severe allergic reaction. About 20 percent of women undergoing this treatment experience slight side effects during its administration. The commonest are headache, chills, and a mild fever. These may be delayed by one or two days.

IVIG must be given about 5 to 7 days before ovulation, and similarly before transfer in an IVF cycle.

IVIG is administered intravenously, slowly over 3 to 4 hours. The first dose is given under medical supervision. Subsequent doses may be given in your own home by a visiting nurse who is trained in the intravenous administration of medicine. IVIG doses are repeated every three to four weeks. How often depends on your reproductive history and the results of blood tests done two weeks after a prior IVIG administration. Usually, no more than three doses are given, but there is no fixed schedule.

"The Second I Received IVIG Treatment, I Became Pregnant"

Elizabeth is beautiful, highly educated, and now in her midthirties. She is married to a man nearly 20 years older than her, and it came as a great shock to this couple that they had to go through such an enormous effort, tragedy, and expense to have their two sons, now aged 7, and 18 months. Elizabeth is forthright in her views about her immune problems and willingness to undergo IVIG treatment. She researched the topic and came to her own conclusions.

❦

I met my husband in my early twenties. We waited a few years before trying for a child. I had three very early miscarriages, all at about 5 to 6 weeks. I had a miscarriage almost every year, but I wasn't really trying very hard to get pregnant, and my regular doctor was dismissive. He said that lots of people have three or so early miscarriages and I should just keep on trying.

Then they began doing a workup on me. I had a laparoscopy, I was put on Clomid, and we began pinpointing the day of ovulation. That time, I got pregnant and although I bled throughout my first trimester, my son was born nine months later. So I had my first child in 1997. When he was 15 months old, we started trying again. I went back on Clomid, but nothing seemed to happen. It was felt best that I should be inseminated via intrauterine insemination (IUI) and I had to persuade my husband to agree at first. We went through seven or eight cycles and my ovaries responded well.

Everything looked fine, but nothing happened. I had another laparoscopy and they found endometriosis, a blocked tube, and a cyst. That led to a lengthy operation as they took the opportunity to clean everything up.

My doctor didn't know why I wasn't conceiving, so he suggested IVF. Again, I had great-looking eggs, so much so that I was worried about a multiple birth. But *nothing*—not even a slight rise in HCG. By now we're onto the 12th cycle and still my embryos are looking good. I was referred to an IVF clinic and went through the next cycle. Everyone was so optimistic about my chances. . . . But even though the embryos looked great—I had nine eggs and seven fertilized, so much so that they were warning me that I might have triplets if they implanted them all—yet three to four days later I wasn't pregnant.

I have a degree in neurobiology. I already knew something about autoimmune diseases. I have a history of them myself, including asthma and Graves disease [which attacks the thyroid]. That was a terrible time, as a graduate student when I thought I was having a nervous breakdown because I was so speedy. It led to my dropping out of law school. I had no idea this might lead to my having miscarriages or being infertile. No doctor had even suggested there might be a link—up to that point.

I started to read up about immunology on the Internet and came into contact with Dr. Scher. I went for immune testing. We found out that my levels of natural killer cells were through the roof, as were my antithyroid antibodies. On the next cycle, I was treated with IVIG and heparin. The IVF worked well and I had three embryos transferred. Amazingly, I got pregnant with twins. Unfortunately, we had another, quite different, run of bad luck in this pregnancy.

Although all was going well, with continued IVIG treatments, in the early days of that December, my older child picked up a virus from nursery school. I got the symptoms too, but we didn't know what it was until too late. It turned out to be scarlet fever. My son and I both became very ill. In my case, I began early contractions. I went to our local hospital, where they did a sonogram, and although we could see the babies' heart rates, I knew something was very wrong. I was bleeding, running a high fever, and in labor. I watched the heart rates falling on the sonogram. I actually saw the babies die on the screen. That was such a devastating experience that it took me about 18 months to get over the infection in my body and trauma of that loss.

When I went back to my doctor to talk about trying to conceive again—I was going to use frozen embryos from the last IVF cycle—it became clear that I needed to give my body a rest. I'd been through hell, I'd had lost about 20 pounds and I had to rest, relax, gain some weight, and get my health back. Then, when I was ready to try, I insisted on having the IVIG treatments. One embryo "took"—and this is my second child. I plan now to go through another whole cycle and try for a daughter. But I'll never do IVF again without doing IVIG.

I admire the doctors who are prepared to stand up for the immunology treatment. If no one was prepared to fight the conservative ways of medicine, we'd never get any changes accepted. It seems to me that it's become quite a political issue. Some doctors refuse to treat women immunologically, even after several failed IVFs. So the women have to go secretly to get the treatment. I've heard doctors say IVIG is like witchcraft. One screamed at his patient and told her to get out of his office, then he slammed the door behind her. But women talk to each other or search on related Internet sites. I get all sorts of phone calls from people who have heard my name or my story.

I'm happy to tell my story, if it helps some other woman or couple out there. I believe I went through all this struggle, the hell of trying to conceive and losing babies, for a reason. Every time I look at my son, I know it was worth it.

❦

"My House Was Like a Fertility Shrine"

Emma is a charming, very slender and athletic-looking woman, now in her midthirties. She and her husband own a beautiful home by the coast, where she works as an interior designer. Like Elizabeth, she did a lot of research before trying IVIG. Upstairs, she proudly showed me the nursery where her two 5½-month-old babies were sleeping in their own rocking chairs. A boy and a girl—the miraculous results of years of tragedy and pain.

❦

We started trying to get pregnant after six months of being married. I didn't focus on it at first, but after two years I wondered what was going on. Something must be wrong? I had just turned 30 and already had spent a whole lot of money on ovulation kits, but nothing was working.

I went to see a fertility doctor locally who started running tests on me. He did a laparoscopy. My insides were perfect! The endometrial lining was normal. I was ovulating properly. My husband's sperm count was normal. This was unexplained infertility. We tried inseminations [IUI] for three cycles, and I was then put on Clomid and inseminations for three more cycles. But I began to develop ovarian cysts, so was taken off the Clomid. The last insemination was the 7th and still there was no pregnancy.

Meanwhile, I had started on a holistic approach, deciding that I should be treating getting pregnant both physically and spiritually. I only ate organic foods and cut down on my exercise, in case I was doing too much, though I always had regular periods.

By now, I was 31 and it was time to start on IVF, so I interviewed a lot of doctors. My first IVF was apparently a success. I responded well to the drugs. The egg retrieval was perfect. In all they got 17 eggs, which is high, and the eggs were all the best; 15 of the embryos survived, with 13 of top quality. The doctor only wanted to put in two embryos because of the danger of multiple births. But nothing happened.

For the second IVF, we were able to do a frozen cycle, using the other embryos. That failed too. By now, I'm getting devastated. I moved onto yoga and meditation. I went to a hypnotherapist, used crystals, and even rubbed African gemstones over me. My house was like a fertility shrine. On the third IVF, amazingly, I became pregnant. This time I was on progesterone and a baby aspirin. We'd seen the heartbeat at 9 weeks, but the fetal growth started to slow down. By 12 weeks, I was warned I might miscarry. The heartbeat was really fading and I had to have a D&C. That was the most devastating time and it was Christmas, too. It's unbelievably traumatic to have gone through three IVFs, finally get pregnant, and then lose the baby.

By now, I knew that something was not right. I decided to

try another doctor. He ran more tests, including a sonogram on my uterus, and did another D&C—he found some of the baby's fetal cells there, so it was good I had that procedure. He also ran the anticardiolipin antibody test on me, and sure enough, it came back positive. My platelets were low and I was suffering hair loss. They were obvious symptoms, but I had experienced my platelets dropping before. It was just put down to stress. No one had associated the condition with pregnancy loss problems, so far.

I began to research it all myself and found that a lot of the autoimmune problems devolve from stress. I had had a very stressful childhood and maybe my body was always in defense mode. It could also be genetic, as I remember an aunt who'd had seven miscarriages and never had any children.

By the time I was ready for my fourth IVF cycle, I decided to work with an acupuncturist too. I also drank a lot of water and took more vitamins and herbs. I was on the baby aspirin, but was also now doing heparin injections three times a day. You have to go to a class to learn how to administer the injections yourself. It's okay, but sometimes you get bruising. But now I'm feeling more prepared. Again they get good eggs and fabulous embryos. Failed.

Now what to do? We did a fifth cycle. Failed. At this point, I was looking into the idea of surrogacy, as my husband refused to adopt. We're Catholic and I could sense he felt this was all a slur on his manhood. Then a friend told me about another immune treatment that is available and the doctors who would use it. I read up about the condition and about IVIG. So, for the sixth IVF, I was given IVIG infusions, still doing the heparin injections and taking baby aspirin. I continued with the yoga and meditation, but by then I gave up the acupuncture, as I had enough needles going in me! I conceived.

With my spiritual approach, I had decided to let go. I felt myself coming very close to God. I would ask him why I had to undergo all this pain. I really began to pray. I prayed to a saint and wore her medallion. I took affirmative seminars and repeated over and over every day, "I'm pregnant with two healthy babies, a boy and girl."

After two infusions of IVIG, then the IVF, a week later my HCG levels were so high they feared I'd have four babies as they had implanted four embryos. In fact, there were three that took hold. I had more IVIG, one embryo lost its heartbeat, but the other two were still growing. In all, I had seven IVIG infusions. The pregnancy progressed, except that by the 8th month I started going into premature labor. I was put on a drug to stop contractions and semi–bed rest. In the 9th month, I was advised to do complete bed rest. Because I seemed to be so stressed, they decided to schedule a C-section at 38 weeks. I'm very thin and carrying twins brings its own complications.

So the twins were born. Now at 5½ months, they're both happy, smiling babies who slept through the night at about 6 weeks. The miracle is that I met the right doctor at that time. I'd do it all again, because I love being a mother. It's such a shame many women only have three attempts at IVF (because that's what insurance covers) and then give up. It really is worth doing everything, and more, that's possible to have your own babies.

❦

"All My Friends Were Having Babies.
Why Couldn't I?"

Nicole offers up an excellent example of what some women are prepared to confront in their desire to beat the problems and have their own babies. Nicole and her husband have two healthy wonderful children: a daughter nearly 5 and a son who is 3. Nicole is now 32. Seven years ago, working as a school social worker while her husband managed his gourmet foods business, they had no way of knowing the problems they were to encounter before having their first child.

❦

I was 25. After three to four months when I didn't get pregnant, I was put on Clomid. Then I became pregnant quite quickly. At 6 weeks, I had my first doctor's visit and everything was fine. But when I went back at 8 weeks, there was no heartbeat. I was told it was a blighted ovum. I had a sonogram and was scheduled for a D&C. It was hard, but the doctor said that 1 in 5 women have an early miscarriage like this. It didn't seem too awful. The advice was to wait a cycle or two, which we did. Then I became pregnant again. I gave myself a home pregnancy test. But I began staining early on. Again we never got to see a heartbeat. They tested my progesterone levels. That night I began getting severe cramps and back pain. I felt that I passed it on the toilet. There was no testing, nothing was done, as the pregnancy was lost.

Now it was becoming more depressing. This was the second one. They say, "It's God's way," but I was getting distressed. I tried a different doctor, who gave me a lot of tests and a blood workup. Again I got pregnant. But this doctor was very callous and didn't want to see me until I was 10 weeks along. We had a huge fight with him and he told me to find another doctor! I went back to the original one and this time we got to see the heartbeat. But then I started bleeding and that was it. This one lasted the longest, we'd made it to 10½ weeks and I really thought I was over the first trimester.

I remember sitting in the hospital crying, waiting for my D&C, with this doctor saying, "Pregnancy is like a game of roulette—one day it will happen." Then my husband was told about another doctor in the city. He made an appointment, which was three months away. That was the day that changed my life. We certainly hadn't reached the point of planning to adopt, but my husband felt he couldn't keep going through these pregnancies anymore. We were young, we wanted our family, it was all too painful. When we met the new doctor, he had such a caring and kind attitude and was much more positive about our chances. He told me how he would manage my next pregnancy. He began with a whole range of tests. There was a mass of blood work. The last D&C meant they could retest the pregnancy tissue, but they didn't find anything wrong. This is what they did find and how they treated it:

- My progesterone level was low, so I was put on progesterone twice a day prior to getting pregnant.
- I have the blood-clotting factor, which means my blood is too thick to pass across the placenta. I was put on heparin twice a day, from ovulation to weeks 37–38 of pregnancy. That meant I had to give myself injections, which leaves some bruising. I also took a baby aspirin every day.

- I was put on Clomid before trying to get pregnant and was inseminated on the right day after ovulation.

Then I became pregnant with my daughter. I carried her to full term and there wasn't a single problem with the pregnancy. I felt wonderful the whole time. I saw my doctor every week until I was about 16 weeks. I had sonograms every week. The two births were expensive, but we both agreed that we were working and could find the money. My husband was great and went to every appointment with me.

I had bought the book about miscarriage, *Preventing Miscarriage: The Good News*. I always remember that line that "miscarriage is something you never forget." The book made me feel so much better, like I wasn't alone. It became my Bible. When the doctor said to me, "You will have your own baby," sounding so confident, that just changed everything. Those two years of miscarrying were so hard. It's really important to have a doctor you can relate to.

I was young, healthy, with no medical disorders or family history of any problems. I remember telling my father, the miscarriages made me feel somehow defective. Now I thank God I have the two children. They have made our house into a home—before that it was just walls.

❡

9

❦

Environmental Factors and
Their Effect on Miscarriage

Environmental factors are often of great concern and a cause of guilt for both parents when they suffer a miscarriage. The mother may feel that it all comes down to something she did or did not do; even a lengthy shopping trip, moving furniture, or an exercise class may be blamed. The father may worry that it was his alcohol consumption or smoking that caused the miscarriage, or the fact that he didn't help enough around the house.

But studies are very inconclusive about specific environmental factors and pregnancy loss or recurrent miscarriage. We cannot really control many factors, other than doing our best to curb certain social habits or known toxins.

Pollution

Very often, after contemplating becoming pregnant or undergoing the stress of conceiving and then losing a baby, we can be overcome not only by grief but also by despair at the world we live in, by the pollution and chemicals with their insidious roles in our lives, by the very water we drink and the air we breathe.

Pregnancy is usually a time of great optimism, buoyed by a renewed confidence in life and humanity, by our faith in the future as we attempt to bring another person into this world. Natural fears about wars, violence, and chemical clouds hovering over us all tend to be dissipated by the sheer magic and joy of the reproductive process.

But when miscarriage casts its shadow, it is not surprising that such issues can lead even the most optimistic of us to a sense of despair. However, as usual, the energy for change tends to come from the women who have found themselves caught by life's unfairness. If nothing else, when you do notice clusters of miscarriages or birth defects, then at least you have the choice: Either you change where you work or where you live or you get out there to lobby for change by the polluters.

Just look at some of the notable pollution hazards in recent times and the effect they have had on world opinion. The terrible accident at the Union Carbide plant at Bhopal, India, led to the release of a cloud of methyl isocyanate gas and possibly cyanide. More than 2000 people were killed immediately. Miscarriages and stillbirths were reported as spin-off effects of the tragedy. The Love Canal disaster, in New York State, came to light when children became mysteriously ill and residents exposed the high rate of miscarriages, stillbirths, and birth defects in the community.

It is very important that we continue to monitor the chemical and radiation levels that have become part of everyday life. There are so many chemicals in everyday use; yet very few have been tested for their effect on pregnancy.

Social Habits That Are Harmful in Pregnancy

Although we can't do much in the short run about the pollutants mentioned above, or about acid rain, there are some toxins we can control.

Cigarette Smoking

One of the best-known hazards in pregnancy, cigarettes affect the whole reproductive process. Smoking tends to decrease the sperm count in men, leads to abnormal sperm, and can promote infertility as well as increase the risk of spontaneous miscarriage. Smoking is harmful as the nicotine crosses the placenta to the fetus and interferes with the blood supply and fetal growth. It can also cause separation of the afterbirth in late pregnancy (abruption). Smokers run double the risk of miscarriage, and those figures increase again with the number of cigarettes smoked daily. Fortunately, smoking can be eliminated at least in our homes, and, hopefully, we can control our exposure to others' smoking at work. Secondhand smoke can also be damaging to the baby's birth weight. Maybe it's time for cars to display yellow signs, in the back windows: Please Don't Smoke, Baby on Board! In many cities, smoking is now banned in public places, and this may help to decrease the impact of this particular habit.

Alcohol

Drinking more than two to three alcoholic drinks a day has been associated with an increase in the rate of miscarriage. But an occasional relaxing glass of wine or beer during pregnancy is probably not significant. The problem is that the exact amount of alcohol that causes harm is not known. So it is safer to avoid alcohol, as it crosses the placenta.

Caffeine

Probably the most widely studied foodstuff, caffeine is included in many food preparations and medicines. It has been shown that if you limit your caffeine consumption to 300 milligrams per day—two fully brewed cups of coffee—there is no association with infertility or miscarriage. So you can be reassured that it is safe to have a wake-up cup of coffee and then one later in the day. Decaffinated coffee is safe, containing 0–3 milligrams of caffeine per cup. Tea has about 35 milligrams per cup. Caffeine has not been associated with any birth defects in the baby.

Workplace Pollutants

Some 60,000 chemicals are used commercially, of which only a handful have ever been tested for their effects on pregnancy. Most researchers, moreover, don't test their effect on miscarriage, but their ability to cause birth defects. Miscarriage is a much more hidden kind of disaster.

Some chemicals, such as DDT, and metals, such as lead, copper, and zinc, may interfere with the implantation of the fetus. Mercury can affect a developing embryo because it can lead to a failure to implant in the uterine lining after fertilization. Some anesthetic gases increase the rate of miscarriage in nurses working in operating rooms. Certain drugs used to fight cancer have also been linked to a high incidence of miscarriages among nurses handling the drugs. However, all such reports are from isolated studies and do not constitute proof.

With the growing number of women in the workplace, our attitude toward such hazards must change. The effect of various chemicals and agents is very difficult to assess during pregnancy, because of the altered physiology of the pregnant woman. For example, the amount of air breathed in pregnancy changes, and the blood volume is increased, which makes the assessment of chemicals' effects even more complex.

Women can be affected if they are working on farms and in gardens, in hospital laboratories and operating rooms; as anesthesiologists, dentists, and dental assistants. All such working women seem to have an increased rate of miscarriage. Women working in chemical industries where rayon, glue, or plastics are made and those who work with radiation or microchips are even more at risk for miscarriage.

If you are working in any of the environments mentioned above you should be encouraged, where feasible, to limit your exposure to the offending chemicals without affecting your position at work. If you are working among such known hazards and cannot be moved to a safer position, you might consider taking a temporary job away from that workplace at least during the first four months of pregnancy, if you can possibly arrange or afford such a break. This also applies in some situations to men; for example, the father's exposure to organic solvents before conception may be harmful to a pregnancy.

Women can be indirectly affected by their partner's exposure to chemicals. He might be bringing lead dust home on his clothes, or traces of chemicals might be detected in his seminal fluid. These chemicals can be absorbed through the vaginal lining. There has been a report that exposure of the father to lead increases his wife's risk of miscarriage. Any man whose partner has undergone more than one miscarriage should inquire at work about the possible reproductive risks to which he is exposed. If these risks are not initially known, then attempts should be made to obtain all the relevant information.

If you are in early pregnancy, or are planning to become pregnant, and you are worried or uncertain about the hazards at your workplace, you should discuss this with your doctor, midwife, or an occupational health physician. You might also inquire from the relevant government agencies or your employers as to the levels of risk. The Occupational Safety and Health Administration (OSHA) issues standards of exposure to lead, mercury, and radiation. You might want to know if you could be removed from a particular working area during pregnancy, or whether you should wear protective clothing. An environmental effect depends also on the amount and duration of exposure, and its timing in your pregnancy.

Here is a list of hotlines you can call if you have concerns.

U.S. Environmental Protection Agency: 202-564-4355;
   http://www.epa.gov
Pregnancy/Environmental Hot Line National Birth
   Defects Center, Kennedy Memorial Hospital, Boston,
   Massachusetts. Will accept calls from practitioners.
   800-322-5014; (inside Massachusetts only) 617-787-
   4957.
Pregnancy Exposure Information Service, University of
   Connecticut Health Center, Farmington; Connecticut
   only: 800-325-5391.
Washington State Poison Control Network, University of
   Washington, Seattle: 800-732-6985; (inside
   Washington only) 206-526-2121.
National Health Information Center: 800-336-4797;
   http://health.gov/NHIC
Food and Drug Administration (FDA): 888-463-6332;
   http://www.fda.gov

VDTs

Well-controlled studies have shown that exposure to video display terminals (VDTs) is not a risk to pregnancy, so normal office work on computers and related machines is quite safe.

Job Stress and Pregnancy

There have been many reports showing that stress in the workplace may affect a pregnancy. For example, one study showed that women lawyers who work very long hours are more than five times as likely to experience stress and three times as likely to undergo miscarriage than a similar group of lawyers who work a more normal 35-hour week. University studies show that long hours of work, standing on your feet all day, or high levels of stress all increase the levels of premature labor.

Such adverse pregnancy complications are on the increase, no doubt due to our changing working habits. One of the most common complications of pregnancy is now premature labor. This may well be due to the fact that great numbers of women have entered the workplace in the past few decades.

There are no magic rules for when a woman should stop working during pregnancy. Your decision should be based on your level of fatigue, the type of work involved, your pregnancy history, and your doctor's opinion. There is no evidence that domestic chores and looking after young children has a similar risk of miscarriage as job-related stress in the workplace. The particular environment, workplace versus home, may play a role in this difference.

Other Hazards to Avoid During Pregnancy

Illicit Drugs

Recreational drugs should *never* be used during pregnancy (or at any other time). They are never pure and may have all manner of harmful effects on the baby (and mother). The baby may even be born with withdrawal symptoms, like an addict, for example, following heroin use.

- *Cocaine:* The drug narrows blood vessels, and pregnancy has been shown to enhance its potency. Besides causing miscarriage, it can lead to congenital abnormalities in the baby, poor fetal growth, and behavioral problems in the child.
- *Amphetamines*: They may cause major growth problems during pregnancy.
- *Marijuana*: While reports of the effects of its use by the parents and on the unborn baby are uncertain, it is safer not to use this drug during pregnancy.

Moving House

The stress and physical labor of moving to a new house or apartment are often linked with miscarriages and premature labor. As I have pointed out previously, neither the psychological or emotional demands of such a move, nor the physical stress of lifting and carrying, will, by themselves, trigger a miscarriage. However, it is advisable, particularly if you have miscarried or have previously suffered from premature labor, to avoid any heavy lifting or unnecessary stress. This is not one of those times to prove how tough you are. Sit back and organize the activity from the sidelines.

The good news about painting and decorating is that paints

no longer contain lead. But if you might be involved in scraping off old paint, let someone else do that. Also try to avoid being in rooms with strong fumes; make sure the windows are open and the rooms are well ventilated. It is advisable to avoid any type of renovation or major remodeling at this time, as there is always a slight risk of breathing in fumes, dust, and particles that would not be good for the pregnancy.

Household Pets

As I have discussed in the chapter on infections, toxoplasmosis can infect the fetus and placenta. It is transmitted by cats, the much-loved pet. The cat is the only host to the infection, but fortunately its incidence is rare in the United States today and is a less serious threat than used to be thought. The parasitic infection may lead to miscarriage, premature labor, stillbirth, or birth defects. Some people have already picked up immunity to toxoplasmosis from living with household pets prior to their pregnancy.

Toxoplasmosis can only be transmitted if you handle the litter tray and come into direct contact with a cat's feces. So if you have to empty the litter tray, *wear rubber gloves.* If at all possible, have someone else do the chore. Other household pets such as dogs, goldfish, and birds do not transmit the infection. Toxoplasmosis can, however, be contracted from eating raw meat or fish.

You may be screened for previous exposure by testing your blood for antibodies, either before conception or when you receive a positive pregnancy test. If you're already pregnant, and you are found to have the disease for the first time, then your pregnancy will be monitored by ultrasound very carefully, to determine if the baby is infected, as there are abnormalities that will reveal themselves. Tests can also be done on the umbilical cord blood and by amniocentesis.

Microwave Ovens

Microwave ovens are a source of radiation, and the Food and Drug Administration (FDA) has established emission standards for any microwave appliance on the domestic market. The permissible limits are 5 milliwatts of radiation per square centimeter, measured at 2 inches from the oven surface. The ovens are safe for home use, whether the user is pregnant or not. Like VDTs, microwaves have become very much established as part of a modern lifestyle. But don't lean against it while chatting on the kitchen phone, for example.

Saunas, Hot Tubs, and Sun Lamps

When your body is subjected to extreme heat over a lengthy period, you may become overheated (hyperthermic), which could adversely affect the fetus. There is no direct link between such usage and miscarriage, but if you are at all concerned, you would be advised against using saunas, steam rooms, or hot tubs while pregnant; or you may be advised to restrict their use to very short periods.

Sun lamps have a strong association with skin cancer, for they expose the body to unusually high levels of ultraviolet radiation. They have not been specifically linked with miscarriage or birth defects. However, as they pose the danger of overheating your body, and as no one knows what the possible long-term effects on the fetus or the pregnancy might be, my advice would be to discontinue their use in pregnancy.

Television

Television rays, even from color televisions, have *not* been shown to be a form of ionizing radiation, so watching television is not harmful, not even sitting close to a television set for long periods.

The only danger would be to your back if you tend to sit slumped for hours on a sofa in front of the set! You would be best advised to sit on a firm chair, so your back is supported, with your feet up on a low stool, to maximize circulation and ease potential lower-back problems. Remember that in pregnancy you should not sit for long periods without frequently getting up and walking about, because of the danger of forming blood clots in the veins of your legs.

Other Factors That Can Affect Your Pregnancy

Advanced Maternal Age

This is an obvious cause of pregnancy problems, but one often overlooked by those trying to begin a family around the age of 40. As a woman passes the age of 35, her chances of miscarrying increase. The reasons are similar to those I have discussed before; they are usually based on chromosomal problems, which arise during cell division with increased frequency in an older woman. The best-known chromosomal problem in older mothers is Down syndrome, caused by the presence of an extra copy of chromosome 21. But there can be extra chromosomes in all pairs except number 1 and the Y chromosome. Because of this, some patients will elect to have chorionic villus sampling or amniocentesis. These are decisions that have to be made by the individual woman or couple in close consultation with her ob/gyn.

It is uncertain exactly how often an older woman miscarries compared to other age groups, as there is the same problem I have alluded to earlier about self-reporting. A younger woman may attribute heavy bleeding one month to a late period, particularly if she did not want to be pregnant, whereas an older woman, if she has previously been pregnant, will more readily recognize the symptoms of pregnancy. Also if she has a strong commitment to being pregnant, she will immediately report a miscarriage to her doctor.

There are also surprisingly high statistics for increased miscarriage in very young mothers, under the age of 18. Why this is so is not known. It could be a reflection of socioeconomic factors; such young women undergoing pregnancy are more likely to have come from lower socioeconomic classes, with poorer nutrition and less availability of health care. Or it could be a reflection of the likelihood of first pregnancies to miscarry more frequently.

Paternal Age

There may be an increased risk of chromosomal abnormalities in a man's sperm as he ages. However, whether this carries an increased risk for chromosomal abnormalities in the baby, as occurs with the mother, is not known. There is currently no recommendation for amniocentesis if the father is older.

Older men's sperm have also been linked to an increase in gene disorders in the child, but, as such cases are extremely rare, we do not know for certain that this is true. There is a test known as the sperm DNA integrity (SDIT), test which tests for faults in the protein (DNA) makeup of the sperm. Defects may lead to fertility problems or an increased miscarriage rate. This test will be considered in cases of unexplained infertility or recurrent miscarriages, particularly if the father has a borderline sperm count.

It has also been questioned whether too many sperm (over 250 million per milliliter) is a cause of miscarriage.

Alcoholism in the father has also been associated with recurrent pregnancy loss, even if the mother is not also an alcoholic. The reason for this is uncertain, but it could be due to stress or a damaging effect on his sperm quality.

Risk of Giving Birth to a Down Syndrome Infant by Maternal Age

The risk of having a baby with Down syndrome increases from age 35. Doctors therefore recommend amniocentesis on pregnant women who are age 35 or older.

MATERNAL AGE	RISK OF DOWN SYNDROME
20	1/1923
21	1/1695
22	1/1538
23	1/1408
24	1/1299
25	1/1205
26	1/1124
27	1/1053
28	1/990
29	1/935
30	1/885
31	1/826
32	1/725
33	1/592
34	1/465
35	1/365
36	1/287
37	1/225
38	1/177
39	1/139
40	1/90
41	1/85
42	1/67
43	1/53
44	1/41
45	1/32
46	1/25
47	1/20
48	1/16
49	1/12

Source: Hook 1978.

Nutrition

The role of nutrition in medicine is becoming more and more important. However, there is no certain evidence that a dietary lack of any single nutrient is a significant cause of miscarriage. At the present time, there is no strong evidence linking even malnutrition to an increased rate of miscarriage. But pregnancy is certainly no time to be dieting, and those women in poorer circumstances, without access to fresh fruits and vegetables, may well run a higher risk of miscarriage.

Women often worry that their nausea, vomiting, or lack of appetite in the first trimester of pregnancy may cause a miscarriage. They fear their nutritional levels are so poor that the baby must surely be starved. In fact, even when the vomiting or morning sickness has reached extreme proportions (known medically as *hyperemesis gravidarum*), requiring hospitalization, there is still no increase in the rate of miscarriage.

Ironically, it is often true that the *more* nauseated you are in early pregnancy, the less chance you will have of miscarrying. Those aggravating symptoms of nausea and the extreme fatigue in the first trimester may be indications that the hormone levels of the pregnancy are adequate.

Folic acid, a B group vitamin, has been shown to be important for normal fetal development, and all women should take at least 400 micrograms on a daily basis before pregnancy. If you have had a previous abnormality of the fetal nervous system in pregnancy, then you should take 4 milligrams of folic acid per day, ideally starting before pregnancy.

Iron intake is also important as there is an increased demand for iron during pregnancy. You will need about 60 milligrams per day, which you will find in a prenatal vitamin tablet.

Is it safe to eat fish in pregnancy?

There is a lot of concern today about whether it is safe to eat fish in pregnancy because of the danger of mercury contamination, which may damage the baby's brain and nervous system.

Eating fish is clearly very healthy for many reasons, such as reducing the risks of heart disease and helping maintain mental and visual function, but because of the mercury exposure risk it is recommended that pregnant women, breast-feeding mothers, and young children avoid eating deepwater fish, which have a high mercury content. These are swordfish, king mackerel, tilefish, and shark. Tuna is also a deepwater fish, but it is widely eaten. Albacore white tuna is higher in mercury content, so you might prefer to eat canned light tuna, as smaller tuna are used for canning and have a lower mercury content.

In place of deepwater fish, you should eat medium-sized fish such as salmon, flounder, and catfish, which are all low in mercury. Because fetal risks depend on the amount of fish eaten and the levels of mercury, it is recommended that pregnant women eat no more than 12 ounces of fish a week (two average meals) and limit albacore tuna to 6 ounces a week.

Exercise and Sporting Activities

There is no evidence that mild to moderate exercise in pregnancy is associated with any harm. Just don't become an Olympic athlete if you weren't one before! And do not engage in very strenuous exercise if you have a medical or obstetric problem. Thirty minutes of moderate exercise a day, most days of the week, is recommended for pregnant women. Regular exercise is encouraged and has many benefits. It may have additional benefits for gestational diabetics.

Only certain women should be discouraged from exercising

vigorously during early pregnancy: those who have suffered more than one miscarriage, those who have had any bleeding or cramping in early pregnancy, and those who have been recommended to take bed rest. If you have a history of premature labor or intrauterine growth retardation, then do reduce your exercise levels in mid-pregnancy.

Exercise and sporting activities, in themselves, will not cause a miscarriage. Aerobics, twisting exercises, jogging, bicycling, and certainly swimming are all safe in normal pregnancies.

Swimming, long known to be one of the safest forms of exercise, comes in for a lot of suspicion during pregnancy. Many women have heard stories that the water may enter the vagina and adversely affect the fetus. This is not true, so unless you have been warned against it for a specific medical reason, swimming is an excellent form of exercise for the pregnant woman.

Competitive sports such as squash and raquetball should be avoided, unless you play them regularly, as the sudden bursts of activity could cause a physical injury. You should also avoid sports where you could fall, such as skiing or horseback riding. Scuba diving must be avoided as the fetus runs the same risk of decompression illness as the diver. Nor should you engage in physical activities at altitudes of more than 6000 feet, though under that is safe. There is no evidence that raising your body temperature by exercising has a harmful effect on the baby.

Physical Trauma

Although many women tend to relate their miscarriages to some event such as heavy lifting, a fall, or even a blow to the abdomen, physical trauma is, in fact, an unlikely cause of miscarriage. And we have all heard tales of young women desperately wishing *not* to be pregnant, going to extremes of jumping from high walls or falling down and still failing to cause a miscarriage.

Early in pregnancy, the bony pelvis shields the uterus from the impact of a blow. Everyday trauma, such as a pelvic examination or sexual intercourse, will *not cause* a miscarriage. It is safe to have a vaginal examination during your pregnancy. Falls, slips, or inadvertent blows to the abdomen are not usually a danger, unless they are extremely severe. The loss of the pregnancy will only ensue if the miscarriage was inevitable anyway. A penetrating injury such as a stab or bullet wound could, of course, harm you and the fetus. But always have a checkup with your doctor after trauma or a fall that has affected your abdomen, so that the pregnancy can be checked.

Prior Induced Abortion

It used to be believed that vaginal termination of pregnancy carried an increased risk of miscarriage in subsequent pregnancies. This is not so. However, when terminations are carried out late in pregnancy and the cervix is forcibly dilated with metal dilators, this can lead to an incompetent cervix and cause a late miscarriage.

Now with very early pregnancy diagnosis possible and the ability to terminate earlier, cervical damage should not be as great a problem. There are also ways of avoiding cervical trauma during procedures. The use of vaginal prostaglandins in tablet or suppository form or laminaria sticks inserted into the cervix the night before an abortion, will encourage slow dilation and thus obviate or decrease the need for mechanical dilators. If you have undergone a previous termination, do not be shy about letting your doctor know so he or she can be aware of the potential for such a problem.

Contraceptive Devices

Many women worry about their use of contraceptive methods prior to becoming pregnant, particularly if there was no real gap between stopping the contraception and conceiving.

If you conceived during the first cycle after you stopped taking birth control pills, you run no greater risk of miscarriage than you would normally. It is only harmful to be taking the pill while you are pregnant.

However, if an intrauterine device is in place when you conceive, then you do run an increased risk of having a miscarriage. The IUD has a higher failure rate than the pill—about 1 out of 100 women using it in one year (versus less than 1 out of 100 women using the pill for a year). If you do become pregnant with an IUD in place, your risk factor increases to 25 out of 100 of having a miscarriage. You will have to discuss with your doctor whether you should have the IUD removed if you are pregnant.

As far as is known, the diaphragm and contraceptive sponge, jelly, gel, and foam have no effect on rates of miscarriage. Spermicides were once implicated in causing chromosome abnormalities, but this research has not been reproduced or shown to be true.

Fertility Drugs

The oral ovulation-inducing agents such as clomiphene citrate or the injectable gonadotrophin drugs are the most commonly used fertility drugs. The risk of miscarriage does increase with their usage, but we don't know if this is linked to the drugs or not, as women with fertility problems have an increased risk of miscarriage to begin with.

If you are taking fertility drugs your doctor will be monitoring your hormone levels closely, so any pregnancy loss will be recorded. Once again, this means that many more early miscarriages are detected and reported. We are not, therefore, sure whether the increased rate reflects a *real* change in the figures or simply more data being recorded.

Progesterone suppositories in the first trimester are often used in pregnancies of women who have previously been infertile or have undergone fertility drug treatment.

DES Exposure

A synthetic estrogen, diethylstilbestrol (DES), was first used on pregnant women in 1948. Because it could control bleeding, it was thought to be useful in certain pregnancy disorders such as threatened miscarriage and premature labor. DES use was discontinued in 1971, so anyone born afterward could not have been exposed to its side effects.

The first reports, in 1977, of its harmful effects on the female offspring of its users were abnormal changes in the vagina, even cancer of the vagina. Subsequent reports also noted that abnormalities of the uterus occurred in 60 percent of girls born to mothers who had used DES. The uterine cavity of a DES daughter could be reduced in size, underdeveloped, or misshapen, typically as a T-shaped uterus. Sometimes adhesions were found inside the uterine cavity. Also, the cervix could be incompetent, or weak. Tubal (ectopic) pregnancies and premature labor are also more common after DES exposure.

These conditions all increased the risk of miscarriage, and the evidence was borne out in studies showing that DES daughters had a higher miscarriage rate than other women. Fortunately, this is a self-limiting condition because DES is no longer used in pregnancy. There are ways to treat all these conditions, except the T-shaped uterus.

If you have had a miscarriage and know your mother took DES, you should have a hysterosalpingogram, an x-ray of your pelvic organs. For this, dye is injected into the cervix so your doctor can look for abnormalities in the uterus or cervix. Further, if your obstetrician knows that you are a DES daughter, he or she

will watch your pregnancies carefully, and your cervix will be frequently checked to see if it is shortening or opening too early.

Surgery During Pregnancy
Whether surgery during pregnancy will *cause* a miscarriage is not
known for certain. If surgery must be performed, the earlier in the
pregnancy the better, particularly during the first trimester. Pelvic
surgery, for removal of a complicated ovarian cyst or an appendix,
are the most frequent emergency situations. If surgery cannot be
avoided, anesthesia must be given so the fetus is well oxygenated.
Anesthetic agents that cause fetal abnormalities in the first
trimester of pregnancy must be avoided. In midtrimester surgery,
drugs such as progesterone or uterine relaxants may be given for
the first two weeks or so following the procedure, and the patient's
uterine contractions will be monitored postoperatively.

It is not definite as to whether surgery causes any harm during
pregnancy, but any elective surgery (one that can be postponed)
should be avoided until after the baby is born or performed before
you become pregnant.

Surgery to remove fibroids at C-section should not be done
unless the fibroid is attached to the surface of the uterus on a stalk
(pedunculated) and can safely be excised.

Acute appendicitis may be difficult to diagnose in pregnancy,
because the pain may not be felt in the typical area due to the altered position of the appendix.

In Vitro Fertilization
In vitro fertilization can carry an increased risk of miscarriage in
the ensuing pregnancy. But as the technique of IVF improves, the
risk factor is decreasing. IVF pregnancies are usually supported in
the early months with progesterone, and you would be monitored
carefully by your doctor.

IVF research is leading to exciting new departures in reproductive medicine. Doctors are better able to evaluate the quality of the sperm and the fertilized ovum prior to implantation, via preimplantation genetic diagnosis (PGD). In itself, this may decrease the number of miscarriages due to abnormal chromosomes in the older mother (over 35).

Artificial Insemination

Artificial insemination by donor (AID) does carry an increased miscarriage rate, and it makes no difference if the insemination is made with fresh or frozen sperm. Interestingly enough, sperm from your partner can cause an even higher rate of miscarriage than sperm from a donor.

Intercourse During Pregnancy

Intercourse during pregnancy may, theoretically, lead to contractions and miscarriage because of the prostaglandins in your husband's seminal fluid. However, there is no definitive evidence, as many couples enjoy intercourse during normal pregnancies with no negative consequences. If you have suffered recurrent miscarriages, you should avoid intercourse until you have passed your prior miscarriage stage. But this does not mean that other physical manifestations of love between you and your partner are contraindicated!

PART THREE

Are You Ready to Try Again?

⚶

10

☙

Why Healthy Grieving Is So Important

Whatever anyone else says, the first thing to bear in mind is that the death of your baby is a profound tragedy. Whether you lose a baby before or shortly after birth, you will be going through an emotionally devastating time. If you miscarried a baby in the very early weeks, your grief may be compounded by the fact that no one else knew you were pregnant, other than your partner and maybe your doctor. And because there were no visible signs, your sadness may be seen by some as inappropriate. "Have another baby quickly" will be their best advice.

Indeed, until recently, miscarriage was treated as an isolated medical condition or "mistake." The fetus would be quickly taken away, and the mother would have no chance to hold or touch it, or even know its sex. You would be put back on the gynecological ward, out of sight and hearing of other babies crying or of mothers holding their new infants. You would be discharged from the hospital and told to see your doctor when next you became pregnant.

This treatment often led to severe psychological reactions, with the mother becoming obsessed with what her body had produced or preoccupied with her guilt and sense of betrayal by her own body.

She may well have spent months, if not years, in a morbid state of unresolved grief, left with her sadness, guilt, fear of inadequacy and failure, struggling alone with these feelings when really the situation was simply out of her control.

Only lately have doctors and allied medical professionals come to appreciate the tremendous emotional impact of a miscarriage; its impact on you as an individual and as a couple, and its impact on family, friends, and other children at home. The American College of Obstetricians and Gynecologists (ACOG) has produced a very helpful pamphlet called *After Your Baby Dies*. You should be given something of this nature, either by your doctor or by the hospital social workers, to read.

At the Mount Sinai Hospital, where I work, the special perinatal social workers who deal with bereaved parents provide a booklet called *Understanding Your Pregnancy Loss: Coping with Miscarriage, Stillbirth or Newborn Death*. It was written and published jointly by the coordinator of the Pregnancy Loss Support Program of the New York section of the National Council of Jewish Women (212-687-5030) and the Mount Sinai Medical Center of New York (212-241-4685).

Why Grieving Is Normal and Healthy

With the loss of a baby, you will never forget that the child was part of you and meant so much to you. Even if he or she had only been a dream in your mind, the baby had already become an important member of your family, an extension of yourselves. The scar left by the loss will never vanish, but you want to come to the point where you can remember your lost baby comfortably and realistically.

You should expect to run through a gamut of emotions: pure grief, sadness, periods of uncontrolled crying, guilt, anger, depression, maybe fear of any ambivalence you felt toward the pregnancy; you may blame yourself, your partner, or even the doctor and the hospital. Also there will be a profound sense of loss that may bring out other losses in your life: a parent, a friend, or even your long years of experience with infertility.

Your first stage in the grieving process will likely be that of *shock and denial*. You may feel stunned and numb, unable to believe what has happened. If it was a very early loss, the pregnancy might now seem unreal, as though you had imagined the whole condition. The emotions of shock and denial actually serve to help us through an overly stressful time, giving us time to come to terms with the reality.

As you develop more awareness and begin to accept the reality, you may begin to develop *somatic complaints*, such as an emptiness in the stomach or chest or a heaviness around the throat. Headaches, sleeping problems, loss of appetite, severe depression—these are all normal reactions. If milk comes into your breasts, you will feel a profound yearning for the baby you never got to hold or feed. Your breasts will ache, along with your heart. If the loss occurred much later in the pregnancy, when you were already used to feeling the baby kicking, it is quite common to go on feeling those lingering sensations. Hearing a baby's cry may bring on terrible crying spurts. Seeing other women with babies can bring out intense anger and pain.

You may well begin to feel afraid that you're going crazy, as your mind struggles to deal with confused feelings and emotions. Somehow, you have to hang on to your sense of self and release the anger and pain.

If it is possible to hold a funeral or memorial service for the dead baby, this may help in bringing on a time of *restitution,* as you get to say good-bye to your lost child. It is important to use the name you were going to call the child, to talk about him or her as a real person. Friends and relatives may find it hard to discuss your loss with you. They will be afraid of bringing back all that grief and of seeing you cry, but if you talk openly and name the baby, then it will be harder for them to ignore what has happened and to utter clichés, such as, "Don't worry, you can always have another."

You don't replace one child with another, just as you'd never replace a family member with a substitute. You must allow yourself to talk about the baby and open up to others.

You may find you don't want to go out of the house and that you avoid social occasions because it is just too difficult to deal with people, their questions, and their insensitivity. At home you will be battling with the void that is now in your life and the terrible awareness of the finality of the loss.

Very likely, you will want to see your doctor to hear reasons and explanations that will help you come to terms with the tragedy. You may still be feeling responsible for the loss. In order to get back to normal daily life, you will need to feel you can share some of that burden in an effort to assuage the guilt.

And slowly, very slowly, you will feel you can embrace the loss and face the future again. At this stage, communication with your partner should be open and nonaccusatory, loving and giving; then maybe you will be ready to try for another baby. But there are other issues involved, too, apart from your inner grieving.

Feelings the Mother Should Expect to Experience

Apart from those feelings connected with a pure sense of grief, there may be other conflicting emotions within.

Loss of self-esteem: How are you going to face the world now? How will you deal with your coworkers, parents, and in-laws, who were all looking forward to this baby?

Guilt and a sense of failure: Is it your fault? Is it a sign of your inadequacy as a woman?

Helplessness: After all, this was out of your control. You ate well, read the right books, tried to lead a healthy life before conception and during the pregnancy. So what went wrong?

Loss of control: This is very hard to deal with, especially if you are used to a level of success and competency in your life and work.

Uncomfortable feelings about your body: Is there something wrong with you? Why did your body betray you? You may feel like a stranger in your own skin, like you no longer understand how your body operates.

Special Feelings If the Miscarriage Occurred in the Early Weeks

This can sometimes prove to be the hardest form of loss, as you might not have even told friends and colleagues yet that you were pregnant. The loss may seem abstract to others, making it hard for them to understand your situation. You may have gone through a horrific experience, with sudden blood loss and painful cramping, and terrifying hours at home. Perhaps an unsympathetic doctor said, "Just go to bed. It will probably be all right." Who else can truly sympathize?

Maybe you miscarried at home alone, on the toilet. All your dreams and hopes flushed cruelly away in a sea of blood. It is hard to banish those images from your mind.

Maybe you carried what you felt was the fetus in a little container, in your bag, on the subway, bus, or in your car, to the doctor's office. What a strange world to have entered.

Special Feelings If the Fetus Was Lost After Week 20

You may have had to experience induction of labor, only to produce a dead baby. Your doctor probably advised you to take medication to help ease the pain of the miscarriage or delivery, and perhaps you can't help feeling guilty that that was what killed your baby (even though it had *no* chance of survival on its own once born so prematurely).

Depending on the attitude of the hospital and nurses, you may have emerged not only empty-armed but seething with anger at the way both you and the dead baby were treated.

If you had been in the hospital or at home on complete bed rest, you may have terrible feelings of failure and frustration at being incapable of producing a child. Lying in bed, not daring to move a fraction in case you set off the miscarriage, can be a terrifying and emotionally devastating experience that few other people will ever undergo.

Doing nothing is the best thing you can do. But how much of nothing is humanly possible?

Were You Able to See and Hold the Baby?

Often parents are afraid to see or hold their dead fetus, because they imagine that the child will look dreadful—perhaps even like a monster. You may find yourself saying, "I'd rather picture the baby in my mind as if she were alive." But it really is best if at all possible to see your baby; otherwise, you might later develop distorted notions of the birth and the real nature of the child. These images can lead to worse feelings, which might crowd out the rather idealized picture you hoped to hold on to.

The fact is that, despite their fears, most mothers and fathers are relieved and pleased when they do see or hold their baby. The hospital nurses or the social worker will bring him or her to you, either dressed in clothes you provided or wrapped in a receiving blanket, maybe wearing a hat to protect the head. The baby's actual appearance, as if asleep, will be far more comforting than any fantasy you could have created.

If you are still undecided, the hospital could take a photograph of the baby. Even if you refuse to see the picture at the time, the hospital will keep that photograph for several months in case you change your mind.

Do you want to hold the baby? Think it over. It can be very helpful just to feel the baby against your body, to give yourself and your partner time to say good-bye. You can let the nurse know if you want her to stay or if you'd prefer to be left alone.

Another very helpful booklet is *When Hello Means Good-bye.* Here is an account they published of a mother and father's time spent with the baby they had just lost.

⚭

Hello, Little Son,

I was so afraid to finally meet you. When you died two days ago inside of me, I was afraid you would not be someone I could recognize and know. Forgive my fears.

The first thing I notice are the birth bruises that any prematurely born infant might have. And there is so much blond hair on your little head. David put a little stocking cap on your head to hide the molding of your skull bones. I know it is a change that comes with death, but also that it's because you are small and were born before your time. Your eyes are closed and puffy. If only you would look up at me. Your mouth is open, with a crimson color to your lips. David thinks you look a lot like your brother. It takes two hands to hold your limp head and body. It is a perfect little body, warm and soft, with all the right number of fingers and toes.

Your color almost looks pink and white except for the bruises and a little vernix on your face and hair. Because everything is so perfect, it is painfully difficult to understand what went wrong. Such a big boy you are—5 pounds and 8 ounces. We supposed you would only be 3 or 4 pounds, coming so soon. And the size of your hands and feet! You don't feel so little as I hold you close.

You are just the right size. There is pain and pleasure in knowing your body, the knees and feet that kicked. We can hold you once, bathe you, dress you. And then we'll say goodbye, keeping only the memory of you and some mementos.

Your body will soon be gone, but the love goes on forever.

⚭

Have You Named the Baby?

Give your baby a name, preferably the one you had been planning for this child all along. Don't "save" that name for your next child, as it rightly belongs to this one. Names are important and will help you talk about this child to others. You will use it when you talk about this baby to your other children or to your family. Memories become firmer when you have a name and face to hold on to.

Keepsakes and Mementos

One of the worst days of your life will be leaving the hospital empty-armed. If your miscarriage was early, you will have only the sense of loss and emptiness inside to see you through. It is hard then to talk about keeping mementos. If the baby was delivered, then you should be able to collect some reminders to take home. Not all hospitals will automatically think of letting you do this, so make a point of asking. For example, you might want to keep

- A lock of hair (though not all babies will be born with hair)
- A set of footprints and handprints
- A birth certificate or certificate issued by the hospital
- A picture of your baby
- The plastic arm bracelet prepared by the hospital to identify your child
- A clipping of paper from the fetal monitor showing a tracing of your baby's heart rate

- A record of the weight, length, head, and chest measurements of your baby
- The receiving blanket your baby was first wrapped in
- A flower from the bouquet brought in by your partner that will have special meaning when pressed into an album

These are only suggestions for you and your partner, at a time when it will be hard to think rationally. You may have other ideas. Be sure to pursue your inner promptings. If you leave the hospital without making your feelings known, without collecting your mementos, you may regret it later.

One of the cruellest ironies is that even though your baby is dead, your need to cradle, nurture, and speak lovingly toward him or her does not diminish. Performing some of these physical and practical tasks may help satisfy a degree of that intense, and unsatisfied, need to care for your baby.

Can Grieving Really Help Overcome the Pain?

Now let me return to the story of Philippa, whom we met briefly in the opening chapter of this book, and how the toll of five miscarriages swept her unwillingly through a door leading to a very different kind of world.

Normally, Philippa is a woman others might envy: tall and beautiful, with a mane of strawberry blonde hair; a kind, loving husband and a bright, pretty daughter of 11. The family lives in an elegant brownstone and they have a country house as well. Artworks adorn their walls, history books their shelves. Philippa involves herself with charity work. It's a comfortable, even privileged existence, except that Philippa has a dark side to her soul. Just recently, she experienced her fifth pregnancy loss late in the second trimester, at around week 23. Each time has been more devastating than the last. Within her story lies much of the material I have been discussing in this chapter. Just how can miscarriage best be handled by the hospital? Does the grieving process really work?

"We Were Able to Cry and to Hold Her"

❦

On my second pregnancy loss at 21 weeks, I asked to see the baby, because I knew it had lived for a few minutes. He was a little boy, strong and beautiful. It shocked me to see him—he was 12 inches long, like a doll, a perfectly formed miniature baby. He looked fine. In fact, I wanted to give him artificial respiration. I just knew he wanted to live. But none of the efforts made could save him. They said he was too young to keep alive. The doctors tried hard to be helpful, but they were really trying in vain.

Eventually, the baby just stopped breathing in my arms. It was a very painful experience. Neither my husband nor I really knew what to do. A nurse came back in and she put a nice blanket around him. Then she took him away; but we never knew where he was taken or buried. I do wish we'd been more prepared, or had someone there to advise us. I would have liked to bury the child, but I just wasn't emotionally ready to start asking such questions.

I lost another pregnancy, again at 21 weeks. Then, on my fourth attempt at pregnancy, although the membranes ruptured at the 24th week, I was given steroids to help mature the baby's lungs in case he was born alive and could be treated.

Well, he was breathing and was born weighing just under 2 pounds, and 14 inches long. He was a very strong little boy, delivered by C-section. Usually C-sections are seldom done at that stage of pregnancy but, if you're trying for viability, it is the least stressful way of delivery. I had had all the risks read out to me: that only 1 in 10 survives at 24 weeks; and I was told about the problems for babies kept in neonatal care units. But my husband and I made the decision because to us 24 weeks seemed so close to the viable age, and I just didn't want to have to go through all this again.

The staff in the neonatal unit were very excited. His brain appeared to be in good shape, because he had not had an intracranial bleed. They fed him little bottles and I pumped my milk. He began to develop a bowel problem, which they corrected surgically. But the anesthesia was very stressful, and after that he developed breathing difficulties. One day he'd be up, the next down. It was agony, a nightmare existence. I'd stayed in the hospital myself for a week, as I was bleeding and unwell. My husband and I visited the neonatal care unit every day. During the last week we were there night and day.

Our poor daughter, who was then 6 years old, was very confused as to what was going on. It really has all been very hard on her. We asked her if she'd like to come and see him, but she was afraid, because she'd heard he had all those tubes wired into him.

He died in his 6th week. We christened him and had him buried ourselves with a nice service. It had been worth the struggle, because there was no brain damage. I met many other mothers in that unit, and the pain they were going through was unbelievable. The nurses were great and the obstetrician was kind and kept calling me. The hospital offered no psychological help, no support. Once a social worker dropped by to see me and said that because she was uncomfortable with death, she'd prefer not to have to deal with me!

I really did feel the lack of someone to talk to after his death. People don't know how to respond. Not that I'd have known before either. I've had friends cross the street rather than have to face me. People preferred to pretend that the baby had never happened. I had someone say to me, "I'm sorry about your little mishap." He was a *person*. We registered his birth. At least the city helped us on that; they sent the birth certificate and at six weeks they sent a death certificate. They acknowledged he was a person. And the insurance company certainly knew it. He came to $40,000 worth of bills! The "little mishap" had quite a dossier.

His death took me a year to get over; not that you're ever really over it. He was my child. I never knew how to explain to people what had happened. You can have very strange reactions that you would not have been able to predict. At home I could not do anything, and certainly could not concentrate. Whatever energy was left had to go to my daughter. We both worked at giving her as much love and understanding as we could. I talked to her and drew pictures of it all, because I was imagining her thoughts must be quite frightening. I also didn't want her to feel that it was her fault. But she seemed mostly concerned about me. Would I ever be normal again? She wanted me back to being the fun-loving mother.

After the baby's death, I just didn't want to become pregnant again. I have a great husband and a lovely daughter. We have a nice life together. So why was I putting myself through all this misery? I was 36 and I'd begun to feel old. Then, I suddenly became pregnant from one night's carelessness, because I hadn't used the diaphragm. I wanted to think it had some meaning, that this was meant to be. I had heard of another team of doctors, so I thought I would give them a try. We felt most encouraged because their attitude was different and they really seemed willing to go that extra mile.

At 7 weeks of this pregnancy, the new doctor put in a suture. I was also put on progesterone and on bed rest. So I took it very easy, though I did have an amniocentesis just in case there were problems. We found out then it was a girl, and we began to feel excited. My daughter named the little girl.

But, at 20 weeks, the membranes were beginning to push through again. I was kept in the hospital and lay there flat on my back, not daring to move or hardly to breathe for three weeks. But the cervix pulled back away from the suture. The membranes burst, and once again I was in labor. It was all over at the end of the 23rd week. I think she died at the time of the birth.

It was so very painful for both of us. I suppose we were prepared to lose her, but we had deluded ourselves as well. They wrapped the baby up for us. She was so pretty and it was nice to be able to see her. You do want to know this is not some "monster" of a child. She had a very tranquil look on her face. We were able to cry and to hold her. Eventually, after we'd been with her for an hour, they took her gently away.

You need that initial time of privacy. Then the social worker at this hospital came by and really talked with us. Also, the doctor did not distance himself. You could see he felt deeply. There was a very real human quality to him that I found helpful. We felt much more supported. We made arrangements to bury her and gave her a little graveside ceremony. She's buried next to her brother.

We'll probably continue trying for a healthy pregnancy.

With our new doctor, and the support of the hospital team, I do feel there is yet hope. But we'll never forget our babies that were part of our lives for such a short time.

❦

Philippa's story brings up other points about the unfortunate experience of multiple losses. If this was a late miscarriage or stillbirth, here are some questions to consider:

- Can the baby be buried, and how do you go about that?
- What can the husband or father do to help?
- How do you cope with the feelings of other siblings?
- How will your body react to the miscarriage?

One of the cruellest aspects of the postmiscarriage experience is that your body exhibits the same kinds of physical changes as those you would have had after the birth of a live full-term baby. Let me give you the hard facts of what you can expect. At least if you are mentally prepared, the pain may be somewhat alleviated.

Your Body Does Not Know the Baby Did Not Survive

If your miscarriage occurred late, it is likely that milk will come into your breasts. This can be painful if you become engorged. Your doctor may prescribe estrogen to take away the milk supply, though using cold compresses and wearing tight bras, with fresh cabbage leaves underneath—this may be an old remedy, but it works—may be all that is necessary.

You will also bleed vaginally. This discharge of blood, called the *lochia,* follows delivery for up to six weeks, depending on how far advanced you were in your pregnancy. If it becomes very heavy, with clots, or painful, or goes on beyond three or four weeks, let your doctor know. Any fever should also be reported to your doctor.

Your first period usually returns four to six weeks following the loss. Once you are menstruating again, it may take three to four cycles to establish your usual flow and regularity.

Postmiscarriage Depression

Even mothers who give birth to full-term, live-born babies are susceptible to postpartum depression. You will be no different, except that in your case, the depression is likely to be worse, as you have suffered real loss and thwarted hopes and desires. The cause of the depression is not known, but bear in mind that powerful hormonal changes are occurring within the body.

The effects of postpartum depression can be quite dramatic for some women, and you should not underestimate your own reaction. When the hormone levels drop in that rapid way, they may also affect your brain hormone levels, which control mood and basic personality. So if you find yourself with wildly fluctuating mood changes, uncontrolled crying, anxiety attacks, strange "crazy" feelings, this might all be part of a typical postpartum response. If your mood slumps into one of despair, your self-esteem is at rock-bottom, and you are afraid of the severity of your own condition, seek help immediately from your doctor or professional counselor.

What Can You Expect Your Partner to Be Feeling?

Fathers who have just experienced miscarriage may tend to be more reluctant to openly express their grief. It is common for the man involved to feel he has to keep control of himself, to be the strong one, so he can support and help his partner through her grief.

Unfortunately for the couple, this type of attitude can be interpreted by the mother as being cold and unfeeling. You might think he didn't really care about the baby. Maybe, you wonder, he didn't really want a baby. Many men say, "I've got to be strong for her," when what they really mean is they don't want to give way to their own emotions or be seen as weak.

Some men will upset their partner even more by making comments such as, "This wasn't really a baby; it's not a great loss. We'll have another one." By talking in this way, they are reinforcing what others may also be saying. The gap between the couple's grief responses can drive a wedge between them, developing perhaps into serious marital problems, especially if there are other domestic pressures.

Even physical violence can emerge, because the man is trying hard to grapple with his own feelings of inadequacy, failure, and unexpressed guilt. He may feel it is his fault, particularly if his wife has had a child by a previous partner. Unable to come to terms with what this means to his masculinity, he may resort to scenes of rage or violence. And, of course, for any couple involved with miscarriage, there are the joint dashed hopes of the "perfect" family, the longed-for happy threesome or foursome. The shared dreams of walks in the park, trips to the baseball game, birthdays, Thanksgivings, and holidays together as a real "family."

Fathers also tend to be left to deal with the practical issues and decisions. If there is to be a burial, the planning may fall on his shoulders. If there are younger siblings at home, he will need to support them through the crisis, while running the household and arranging visits to the hospital. At the same time he will have his own grief to deal with.

One of the most painful ironies a father may have to confront will be receiving the hospital bills for this birth that has not brought them the much-wanted baby.

Helping Your Other Children Cope with the Loss

You should consult your pediatrician on how best to help siblings come to terms with what has happened. You might instinctively feel you want to protect your other children from the sadness of this lost pregnancy or from the death of an infant. But avoiding discussion may make your child at home feel more, not less, upset. Your child will be sensitive to your moods anyway, and will wonder why he or she has been left out. A simple, honest explanation that reassures them of their own safety is the most helpful.

Younger children can feel guilt, as Philippa described. For example, the child may have been secretly wishing the new baby wouldn't take up so much of Mommy's time, and the sudden death may make her feel she has brought this about.

The way children talk about or express their feelings depends on their age and stage of development. For example, a 5-year-old was told Mommy was pregnant, that a little sister or brother was growing in her tummy. When he heard that the baby was gone, he asked his mother *where* the baby had gone. The mother replied that the hospital would be looking after the baby. A year later, when they were driving by the hospital, the little boy suddenly said, "Can we go and see the baby now?"

Many parents find it easier to wait for the child to bring up the subject, worrying about his or her response to the idea of death. Certainly you don't have to go into detail about death, but it is best to approach the subject yourself, and then not to use explanations like, "We lost the baby." To a 3-year-old, that might mean it will soon be found, or that you might also "lose" him or her. Similarly, don't say, "The baby was sick and died," or "The baby is sleeping." Such words could play into the imagination of a young child who may then fear going to sleep or getting sick. You will have to reassure your young child that nothing he did or thought made the baby die.

With a child older than 4 years, you should encourage looking together at a photograph of the baby. If the child is about 8 years old and you are going to have a funeral, you might want to let the child come along.

Remember, as Philippa mentioned, older children living through the experiences of multiple miscarriages may fear losing *you,* that something will happen to you.

Watching you rush to the emergency room several times, or being hospitalized, and witnessing your tears, sadness, and depression can be hard on them. Try to be as positive in your discussion of birth and death as possible.

How Family and Friends Can Help

Family and friends should be encouraged to take an active, helpful role. Both you and your husband will be going through emotional turmoil, during which time it is hard to make decisions. You need one friend or family member to take over the burden of making phone calls or sending out cards to those who need to know the news. If you try to do this, you will only become upset each time you begin a new phone conversation. Ask someone to take over that role for you.

Professional counseling or a support group can also help to relieve your pain, guilt, and depression and help you understand and accept what has happened. You may wish to seek counseling just for yourself, for both you and your partner, or, if another child is seriously disturbed, for the whole family. Think about counseling if you find, for example, that (1) you are *stuck* in one phase of the grief process, so that you are having trouble working through certain problems alone or with your partner; or (2) severe physical or emotional problems are preventing you from functioning, such as being able to return to work, to care about your health and appearance, from sleeping, or getting out of bed in the morning. (See the Resources section for a list of support groups or related websites.)

Arranging a Funeral or Memorial Service

Immediately following a miscarriage, parents are usually still in shock from their unexpected loss. But if the baby was lost around week 15 or later, they may have to decide whether they want a funeral or another type of ceremony. Your doctor, nurse, or social worker will speak with you about these matters. You may choose to talk with your local clergy or with the hospital chaplain of your faith about the loss and about burial practices and rituals, as they vary among different denominations.

If your baby was miscarried in the early weeks, so there can be no burial, you may wish to create a ritual or a memorial service to say good-bye to the child. For some parents, it can be a great comfort to have family and friends acknowledge the life and death of their baby and to express their sorrow at a special service.

As Your Feelings Gradually Return to Normal

There will be days when you'll wonder if your mood and sense of optimism will ever return. For most of us it does. And then you may slowly begin to feel ready to start again, with a new pregnancy. The following passage, which is also from the booklet *When Hello Means Good-bye,* shows how that change does slowly take place.

❧

"Where is your baby?" Until yesterday, the joyful, expectant look that accompanied the question started me crying. It's only today, one month later, that I can reply, with peace in my heart, that our baby is gone, that he died before he was born.

Physically I am healed. My body has forgotten the pregnancy, but my mind is still letting go. The empty, sad feelings have lessened, and there are more times when it is possible to laugh or just to feel at peace. Getting to sleep at night is easier now than it was that first week. But fixing meals and eating them is still a chore. I've learned that eating sugar or consuming alcoholic beverages or skipping meals can bring my mood crashing to the floor. The anger I didn't feel so much at first now comes out suddenly in the form of irritability with David and the kids, especially when I am tired. Fortunately, I have taken time off from work to just take care of myself.

Both writing down how I feel in my journal and exercising regularly help me to get through the day without being overwhelmed by my feelings of depression and anger. I talk for hours with friends, totally unaware of the time passing. Right now there is only one reality, loss and grief. The greeting card companies and people in general expect that each day will get a little easier and a little brighter for people in my situation. But that's not exactly how grief works. For me the days are unpredictable. Some days it seems like every woman I see is pregnant or carrying a newborn baby. *It's just so unfair.* On other days I remember vividly what Tony looked like, and I feel again the love and peace we shared at his birth.

Loving Tony has brought David and me closer. I am so grateful we can share this burden. I am told that time will heal the grief, but now I know that it is taking the time to grieve that heals.

☙

Are You Ready to Try for Another Pregnancy?

As I mentioned in Chapter 1, the only medical factor to consider is the presence of pregnancy hormones, which could produce a false-positive pregnancy test until about the third week after a miscarriage. It is advisable, therefore, to wait until you have had your next period, sometime in the following four to six weeks, after which the pregnancy hormones will have disappeared. Then if you feel emotionally ready, you can try to conceive. Remember, there is no medically indicated waiting period, as it has been shown that a pregnancy conceived shortly after miscarriage is at no greater risk of miscarrying or being abnormal.

As for the psychological factors I have been discussing, only you as a couple can evaluate them. Some researchers point out that if you conceive very quickly, you may find yourself still going through intense grieving for the lost baby—for example, around the time of its expected due date—at a time when you should be making a healthy relationship with the next baby.

You could ask yourselves questions like those that follow to see whether you are in fact ready to conceive again.

- How do you feel about holding or seeing other people's babies?
- What do you feel when you see other pregnant women?
- What will it be like for you to return to the same hospital?
- What do you feel like walking through the baby department in stores?
- Can you sense a difference between how you were feeling a month after your miscarriage and how you are feeling now?
- Do you have more control over the unexpected bouts of weepiness?
- Have you sought support or really been able to talk over your feelings with someone who understands?

That's not to say you have to be completely free of pain, anger, or resentment before planning another pregnancy. But it is advisable to check in with yourself about your levels of anxiety and sadness, and feel that they are at a reasonable level before trying again.

Coping with the Next Pregnancy

The next pregnancy will be a time of very high anxiety, especially in getting past that particular week (or those different weeks) when you suffered your loss or losses. You will feel panicky and there will be agonizing moments in the bathroom when you check yourself for signs of staining or worry that gas pains are cramping.

I would like to offer the following advice to ease you through this as painlessly as possible:

1. Talk to your doctor. Make sure he or she is prepared to listen to your fears, and to talk to you honestly about the problems, and hope, involved.
2. Request ultrasound scans to reassure yourself at regular intervals that the baby is all right, even if the scans are not required for medical reasons.

You may want to talk about a future pregnancy with a social worker or psychotherapist so that you can come to some compromise with yourself about what is reasonable in terms of anxiety levels. You do not want to face nine months of constant worrying. Some doctors advise setting aside a certain hour each day for worry. Then try and put the panic to one side for the rest of the day. Be prepared to rest more, even to start complete bed rest if it is felt advisable.

Think as positively as possible. Concentrate on doing everything possible to produce a healthy baby. Your doctor is aware of all the latest information, and you can rely on his or her medical skill. Many, many women—as you have read in this book—do come out of the long dark tunnel, even after several miscarriages, with a beautiful, healthy, full-term baby.

11

꙰

What Should You Expect
During Your Next Pregnancy?

It has been shown that recurrent pregnancy loss, whether from repeat miscarriages, unexplained infertility, or failed IVF, is associated with other problems that can arise during a pregnancy, including ectopic pregnancy, preterm birth, pre-eclampsia, fetal growth retardation, stillbirth, and an increased chance of delivery by C-section or forceps at the time of birth. So the next time you become pregnant, you will be managed as a high-risk patient. There is also concern for possible chromosomal problems in patients with recurrent miscarriages, and you should probably undergo genetics testing by amniocentesis or CVS during the pregnancy.

You will be monitored early on, because of the increased risk of ectopic pregnancy. This is done by measuring pregnancy hormone levels and repeating the test every 48 hours to see that it doubles in this period. At the same time, it would be helpful to measure the progesterone level, as this would usually be very low in a tubal pregnancy. Once HCG levels have reached between 3000 and 5000 units, a pelvic ultrasound scan will confirm that the pregnancy is in the correct place inside the womb. (If not, this may indicate an ectopic pregnancy.) An ultrasound scan can show a sac in the uterus 10 days after a missed period, also helping to exclude an ectopic pregnancy. It will also exclude a molar pregnancy. This is a rare tumor of pregnancy, but one that is more common in women with recurrent miscarriage. It can be successfully treated.

As soon as you suspect that you are pregnant, you should contact your doctor. My maxim is "Difficult at the beginning and difficult at the end," to remind doctors of the importance of frequent monitoring in women who have previously lost several pregnancies.

How will your pregnancy be managed if you are currently being treated for recurrent miscarriage? The methods of treatment will depend on the causes that have been found, although the treatment for a new pregnancy will actually have begun before you even try to conceive. Any treatment you are currently receiving will be continued into the pregnancy. You should be taking a prescription prenatal vitamin, containing 1 milligram of folic acid. You may have been prescribed an extra amount of folic acid if you are known to have an abnormal blood-clotting factor, such as a raised homocysteine level, or if you have had an abnormal fetus, especially one with a brain or spinal defect.

So if you think you might be pregnant it is important that you contact your doctor immediately and have your HCG and progesterone levels tested, to reassure you that the embryo has implanted in the uterus.

As a high-risk pregnancy, you will be seen by your doctor at least every two weeks throughout the pregnancy, rather than the usual four weeks. Besides being important medically, this provides psychological well-being for the couple (though frequent visits may induce anxiety for some). In early pregnancy, you might be seen every week, aside from visits for blood tests. If you need the extra reassurance, I'm sure your doctor will be happy to let you listen to the fetal heartbeat or have regular ultrasound scans to see it. In fact, you should have ready access to your doctor's office to talk over any concerns. In some cases, reassurance will counter the negative effects of too much stress and anxiety. So don't hesitate to ask for this extra level of support.

You should rest as much as possible in early pregnancy. This rest mimics what nature intends as it gives the implanting embryo time to take a secure hold in the womb. In normal pregnancy, women tend to feel very tired in the first trimester and generally lacking in energy. This is nature's way of telling you to take it easy, in all probability to maximize the blood flow to the new pregnancy.

Of course, you can do a reasonable amount. I am not suggesting every woman has to take bed rest—unless specifically advised—but if possible, try to rest for half a day or maybe three hours a day during this early stage. It should make you feel better and reassure you that you are doing everything possible to support the pregnancy. Try not to rush around, commute for long hours, or burn the candle at both ends.

It is also a good idea to abstain from sexual intercourse until you are past the miscarrying stage; the hormone prostaglandin in seminal fluid can bring on a miscarriage (but only if you are prone to that causal effect). Abstinence also reduces the risk of infection being introduced into the womb.

In most cases, exercise and intercourse can be resumed after week 12 of pregnancy, depending on your past history, as the most dangerous time for a threatened miscarriage is in this first trimester.

Apart from this extra advice, you will continue receiving the normal routine pregnancy information. For example: replace aspirin with Tylenol; take your prenatal vitamins; limit yourself to two cups of coffee a day; cut out smoking and alcohol—except perhaps for the occasional drink on a special occasion.

You might have been put on progesterone vaginal suppositories or, if you underwent IVF, an intramuscular injection of progesterone. If so, this treatment should be continued to at least weeks 12 to 14 of pregnancy, as natural progesterone has a lot of positive benefits for you. It aids the immune acceptance by your body of the pregnancy and provides nutritional support by thickening the lining of the womb to nourish the embryo. It also reduces levels of prostaglandins that can cause inflammation and possibly lead to miscarriage. Discuss these matters carefully with your doctor. Once you are off intramuscular progesterone shots, I recommend using progesterone as a vaginal suppository as this delivers higher levels to the womb itself than the injections, which give higher blood levels. The pregnancy maintenance dose is 200 milligrams of vaginal progesterone suppositories, inserted three times daily.

You will receive the routine prenatal blood tests, of course: blood group; immunity to rubella and toxoplasmosis; tests for any sexually transmitted diseases, including HIV; thyroid function studies; and additional testing according to your needs. Certain genetic screening tests will also be done, depending on your ethnic background, for example, for cystic fibrosis and Tay-Sachs. New screening tests are constantly being discovered and your doctor will tell you about them.

If you are going to be over 35 when the baby is due, you will be offered chromosomal testing, for example, amniocentesis and chorionic villus sampling. If you have had recurrent miscarriages, where the incidence of abnormal chromosomes may be higher, this will be even more vital. At this stage, if you have previously miscarried several times, or have gone through infertility or become pregnant following IVF, the decision as to which method of chromosome testing is to be used is difficult. You may be hesitant to have an invasive test such as CVS or amniocentesis because of the miscarriage risk (though it is small), and might prefer to do a first-trimester screening procedure, which does not put the pregnancy at risk.

The new *nuchal translucency measurement test* is performed by ultrasound, measuring an echo-free area at the back of the fetal neck and is usually accompanied by blood testing. It does not carry a risk of miscarriage, but is only around 90 percent accurate. However, it is performed before week 14, ideally at 11 weeks, which is before the time amniocentesis is performed (16 weeks), so that if the results are normal, then you will have that extra reassurance. If there are indications of abnormality on that test, however, you might then decide to go ahead with CVS or later amniocentesis.

If you are over 35, besides chromosomal abnormalities, you are also at increased risk of developing certain medical conditions such as gestational diabetes, pre-eclampsia, and high blood pressure. You will be watched carefully for the onset of any such conditions.

Routine *alpha-fetoprotein (AFP) screening*, which is done via a blood test from 16 weeks, could indicate the necessity to undergo amniocentesis if the result is reported as low. When the test result is high, it may indicate spina bifida, but then the test is usually repeated, as it does produce false positives. A low result may mean chromosomal problems; in such cases the test will not be repeated and amniocentesis will be recommended.

A *high-resolution ultrasound scan* is carried out from 18 to 20 weeks to assess the detailed anatomy of the baby. This can be a pleasant experience for you and your husband, and you may even find out the sex of your baby at this time, if you want to know. It can also give clues as to whether you should undergo amniocentesis, as some anatomical abnormalities are found in certain chromosome disorders.

If your prior pregnancy loss occurred because of an incompetent cervix, you will probably go into the hospital to have a *cervical stitch* put in around week 12. The stitch is removed in your doctor's office around 36 weeks, once your baby is mature.

During later pregnancy, you must watch for *signs and symptoms of premature labor.* These are vaginal bleeding; a heavy mucus discharge, suggesting that the plug in the cervix has been expelled; frequent uterine contractions; severe low backache; or any hint of leakage of amniotic fluid. You must report these signs immediately to your doctor.

There are new ways of predicting the onset of premature labor, such as testing for a protein called *fetal fibronectin (FFN).* Your doctor will take a swab from the top of the vagina, behind the cervix, every two weeks from weeks 22 to 32, as necessary. This will be performed if you are at increased risk for premature labor; for example, if you have a history of premature labor or are having a twin or triplet pregnancy. The result is obtained within 24 hours; if the test is normal, it means you won't go into labor for at least two weeks, which will be very reassuring.

It may be necessary to do a *vaginal culture* at intervals for bacterial vaginosis (BV), an infection that can encourage premature labor and, if found, be treated with antibiotics. Urine cultures are also done repeatedly for the same reason.

If labor or excess contractions start at less than 36 weeks of pregnancy, your doctor will hospitalize you for treatment to stop the uterine contractions, as they could lead to premature birth.

After your condition is stabilized, you may remain in the hospital for a period of time for observation, or your doctor may consider sending you home with instructions to return if symptoms of preterm labor occur again. When you are discharged from the hospital, your doctor may also prescribe *home uterine activity monitoring (HUAM),* which allows the contractions of your uterus to be monitored, at least twice a day at home, as the signal is transmitted over the phone line to a nursing station for review. The contraction monitoring device you would use at home is similar to the monitors used in the hospital. If anything on the HUAM looks suspicious, the monitoring nurse will talk with you and call your doctor or tell you to go to the hospital for evaluation.

This service is provided by a national home obstetric care company called Matria Healthcare and can be very reassuring to expectant parents. It means you are not left alone at home, with the responsibility of wondering what to make of contractions, or being afraid you will miss signs of premature labor, which, after all, is one of the commonest pregnancy complications today.

A new effective preventative approach when the mother has a history of prior preterm birth is the use of a form of progesterone known as 17P (17alpha-hydroxy progesterone caproate). This drug relaxes the uterine muscle and makes the uterus less able to contract. It is given weekly by intramuscular injection commencing at 16 to 20 weeks and continuing up to week 36 of pregnancy.

If you do go into premature labor, you must be hospitalized and be treated very rigorously.

When we are considering the management of pregnancy, after treatment for recurrent miscarriages or repeated failed IVF, we have to consider the cause of the problem and the types of treatment available very carefully.

If you conceive following IVF, then there is a greater incidence of miscarriage and a higher risk of ectopic pregnancy and of multiple pregnancies. This means more frequent prenatal visits to watch out for these conditions, which will require special care if they occur, for example, removing a tubal pregnancy with drugs or surgery, and preventing premature labor with a multiple pregnancy.

If the baby is not growing well during your pregnancy (this is called growth retardation), you may be put on bed rest, particularly lying on your side (the left side is better for blood flow to baby than the right side). This will be supported by frequent non-stress tests and biophysical profiles through ultrasound to ensure that the placenta is providing adequate oxygen and nutrition to the baby. You may need to be induced once the baby is mature and not be allowed to go the full 40 weeks.

If your pregnancy is high-risk and you go into labor or your water breaks, you must be admitted to the hospital immediately for continuous fetal heart rate monitoring. In such pregnancies, there is a strong chance that the baby will be delivered by C-section (the rate is up to 60 percent).

Specific Therapies or Treatments That May Be Prescribed

Intravenous Immune Globulin

If you become pregnant after repeated miscarriages or failed IVF procedures, you should expect your doctor to suggest immune testing, for which treatments, including IVIG and heparin, are available if the tests are abnormal. You should not be subjected to multiple repeat IVF procedures, at enormous financial, physical, and emotional cost, without these tests being done.

If you are to receive IVIG, ideally it should be started preconceptually or pretransfer and then continued every three to four weeks, once you become pregnant. Before you receive the first dose, you must have two blood tests. One is for total IgA: if you lack this in your blood, then you cannot receive IVIG (this affects 1 in 800 women). The other is for serum creatinine to ensure your kidney function is normal.

The first dose must be given under medical supervision, in your doctor's office or the hospital. But subsequent doses can be administered at home by a nursing service. How many doses you receive will depend on the reasons for being given the treatment. For example, for raised NK cells, it depends on how you respond, as assessed by the results of a blood test two weeks after a treatment dose. If, however, you are receiving the IVIG for raised auto-antibodies, such as antithyroid antibodies or antiphospholipid antibodies, it is often continued until later in the pregnancy. If you have a condition such as lupus or autoimmune hepatitis, it may be continued throughout your pregnancy.

Remember, IVIG is not approved for pregnancy and fertility usage by the FDA. But as it is a safe drug with no long-term side effects, it is used "off-label" in this way. However, you will have to be educated about IVIG before you decide to go ahead with what is regarded as experimental treatment.

Heparin

You might be given heparin to treat factors that interfere with blood flow. This aids in the penetration of the embryo into the uterine wall during implantation, helping growth of the fetus. Heparin is either given twice daily (soluble heparin) or once a day (low-molecular-weight heparin, as Lovenox) by subcutaneous injection. Heparin is safe in pregnancy and does not cross the placenta. Nevertheless, every month your clotting functions and blood count (including platelets) will be monitored. Heparin does increase the risk of bone thinning, so you must be sure to take at least 1500 milligrams of calcium and 400 units of vitamin D daily to counter this risk. You would usually continue heparin to about week 35 of pregnancy. You will also likely be taking a baby aspirin to week 36. You would not want to go into labor while on heparin or aspirin, as this may preclude your receiving a spinal or epidural anesthetic.

As it may cause bruising of the skin, heparin is usually injected in a less visible place, such as the lower abdomen. Remember, this is prophylactic heparin (not therapeutic high-dose heparin) and it should not cause bleeding, except for possible slight bruising at the site of the injection.

Prednisone or Dexamethasone

You may have been put on either Prednisone or Dexamethasone at the start of your cycle, at about day 5. These drugs are given to lower levels of antibodies that may be harmful. They are given in low dosage and are usually stopped at about weeks 9–10 of pregnancy. Prednisone has been associated with premature labor and gestational diabetes and is therefore always discontinued before week 20. When these two drugs are to be stopped, your doctor will instruct you to taper off gradually.

Natural Progesterone

Progesterone is the most important pregnancy hormone. It prepares the womb lining for receiving the embryo by ensuring sufficient nutrition and by helping the mother's body to adapt to the embryo immunologically, allowing the pregnancy to implant and proceed successfully. It is usually given as an injection or vaginal suppository three to four days after ovulation, or on the day after transfer in an IVF cycle. Once pregnancy is diagnosed, it is usually continued until the end of the first trimester of pregnancy, around 12 to 14 weeks.

Glucophage

Glucophage (Metformin) is used to treat polycystic ovarian syndrome (PCOS) associated with insulin resistance. It helps spontaneous ovulation and conception to occur in those patients, being started by mouth once the condition is diagnosed, and it can be continued throughout pregnancy. It may also improve egg quality, which is important in IVF cycles. Glucophage has not been associated with an increase in birth defects. Of course, as with so many treatments used in pregnancy, more studies need to be done. The risk-benefit ratio must always be taken into account when using medications, so you must discuss this with your doctor.

Late-Pregnancy Treatments

Pre-eclampsia, intrauterine growth retardation, gestational diabetes, premature labor, premature rupture of the membranes, and placental abruption (separation) must all be carefully watched for and treated. Close monitoring of the baby in late pregnancy with ultrasound, biophysical profiles, fetal weight measurements by ultrasound, and nonstress testing every three to four days are all employed. The doctor cannot relax his or her surveillance once you are pregnant or past your miscarrying stage. Interestingly, patients who have received heparin during their pregnancy often deliver two to three weeks before term, at around 37 to 38 weeks. You may also have to be induced before full term if there are signs of growth retardation or some other medical condition such as high blood pressure.

"I Just Don't Believe I'd Have Gotten Where I Am Now If I Hadn't Decided to Use the IVIG"

Sarah is an orthodox Jewess who was married when she was 24 and expected to have a large family. Being young, she and her husband decided to wait a year or two before trying for a baby.

❦

When we did start, four years ago, I was sort of taken aback that I didn't get pregnant immediately. In fact, it took about three months and already I was getting crazy. I had my first doctor's visit and saw the heartbeat at around 6 weeks. It looked great but, at the end of the first trimester, suddenly there was no heartbeat. I had to have a D&C, and, even then, I was devastated. That summer I was so depressed. My obstetrician said to wait a month before trying to get pregnant again and it happened in October. He said he'd watch me more carefully. I was allowed to have visits every two weeks. I was nervous and anxious, but he said it was quite normal to have one early miscarriage.

When I went back at 8 weeks, there was no heartbeat. I was screaming with hysterics. But again the doctor said it was normal and to keep on trying. I had a few tests done and everything appeared normal. By now, I was totally nonfunctioning. I couldn't meet up with friends who had babies. I even found it hard to go to synagogue. My mother said I should see a therapist, as I was just not right. Then one day I went into a large bookstore and looked up miscarriage. I came across the first edition of *Preventing Miscarriage: The Good News*. That was the moment that began to change my life. The book was like my Bible. I read it from cover to cover the first night and kept it on my night table.

I found a new obstetrician, in the city, never minding the cost. He did all the routine blood work and immune tests. The results showed that I have high NK cells and also the blood-clotting factor. We had some immune treatment and I became pregnant again, but it wasn't right as I started staining. The doctor did a sonogram and there was an empty pregnancy sac—it was a blighted ovum. The next pregnancy was ectopic. I had to have surgery and lost my right fallopian tube. So now it seemed to me I only had half the chance to get pregnant. You can imagine how I was feeling!

I joined an IVF program. I was put on Clomid and we tried IUI, but that didn't work. Then we were ready for our first IVF cycle. I hyperstimulated and produced too many eggs and so we had to stop. Knowing the arguments over whether to use IVIG or not, I decided I might go for treatment, even though the IVF obstetrician was against it. I'd met other women who were doing the same. They all seemed to know so much—they'd researched it very thoroughly.

For the next pregnancy, I was put on blood thinners and baby aspirin. My first sonogram showed I'd conceived twins. I was so happy! But that night, when I went to the toilet, it was full of blood. I was crazed. The doctor said that I'd lost one baby—out of what turned out to have been triplets. I still had twins in the womb and there was a healthy heartbeat. It felt as though God had given me back my life. I was having weekly sonograms, but one of the twins' heartbeats became very slow and it died.

By now, I was 26 and this was my first chance at having a live baby. Even though IVIG was going to be very expensive, we decided to go with it. I had three treatments of IVIG and after that it was a normal pregnancy. My baby was a girl and she was born at a healthy 9 pounds 2 ounces. There I was, after not being able to hold a pregnancy at all, delivering a healthy 9-pound baby! I just don't believe I'd have gotten where I am now if I hadn't decided to use the IVIG. I was maybe more scared of it than other women I've met. But my desperation to have a baby overrode the fears.

Then I wanted to get pregnant again. This time I had IVIG before the egg retrieval and in all had about six IVIG treatments (we've spent $7500 on IVIG on this pregnancy). I'm so excited. I'm due in a couple of months' time and my first baby is now 17 months old. We'll do it all again, too. I really do want a relatively large family. We'll just have to take out loans!

"I Did a Lot of Research Then and Went to See Many Doctors"

Joanne is an attractive and thoughtful woman whose first child, born nine years ago, was a perfectly normal uncomplicated pregnancy and birth. She was an advertising executive, but with the miscarriages and then going through the IVF program, she decided to give up her full-time career to concentrate on becoming a mother and developing her writing talent.

It was always easy to get pregnant. The first baby was born when I was 31. An easy pregnancy and vaginal delivery. He was a colicky baby, but I became pregnant again when he was 18 months. I miscarried at 11 weeks. I wasn't high-risk, being just 32, but there wasn't a heartbeat. I had a D&C, no chromosome testing or anything like that. It was all quite uneventful. Sad, but not desperate, as I was relatively young. A year later, I became pregnant again. This time, I got to 20 weeks, but when I was hanging drapes, I stretched a little too much and started to bleed. In fact, I was bleeding so heavily that I was hemorrhaging. It was the day of the New York City marathon and I had a hard time getting across the city to the hospital. It was pretty scary.

Once in the hospital, they located a heartbeat and I was sent home to try and save the baby through bed rest. I lay there for a few weeks but, at 23 weeks, we decided to get different opinions. We found out that the placenta had abrupted. I could have died if it ruptured. I remember looking around the neonatal unit at all the tiny preemie babies. We made a very difficult decision—to terminate that pregnancy—as the risk was very high, either to my health, or that the baby would be born dangerously early. It was termed a late abortion and was horrible. In no way was that a frivolous decision. I had to go into labor, using laminaria to soften the cervix. The fetus, a boy, was born dead, weighing just 1 pound. They did a million tests of the fetus and on me. My NK cells were slightly elevated and it was also thought I had an autoimmune condition.

I did a lot of research then and went to see many doctors. When I was younger, I wanted to go to medical school so I had no problem researching these topics. Although I'd never had a problem getting pregnant, I decided to take Clomid. I became pregnant again, then lost a third one. This time it was a blighted ovum. Then there was a fourth. Again taking Clomid, became pregnant, but on the second doctor's visit there was no heartbeat and I had to have a D&C.

By now I was becoming obsessed. Why was I not having a second baby? My elder child was 3 years old. I became determined to find out what was going on. On reading it all up, on the Internet and in books, I decided that for the next pregnancy I'd go through the IVF program and would take IVIG for the immune problems, progesterone, and baby aspirin.

With my first attempt at IVF, they harvested nine eggs and gave me back three embryos. I decided to have them all implanted, even though I knew there was a danger either for me or for the potential triplets. However, a scan showed that one was not faring well, so we came to a decision to have a selective termination of two of the fetuses. It was a difficult decision, but the prognosis for a live birth of one baby was more positive than for twins or triplets.

The pregnancy then went ahead fairly normally. And my little girl is now 5 years old. She's incredibly articulate, funny, and confident. I just can't see that she would have the same personality if she was one of twins. I wouldn't have minded twins if I'd felt sure that it would be safe and that I would have carried them healthily to term. Multiple births are very common now, in New York City at least. So many women take fertility drugs and go through IVF, you just see double and triple buggies wherever you go. In my 5-year-old's class, out of 60 kids, there are three sets of twins and one of triplets. That's a very high proportion.

Did I need all that medical intervention in the end? Who can say? I didn't mind taking the IVIG at all. Okay, it's a blood product, but it's safe and controlled. The irony is that since then, I've had a third baby, conceived and born the natural way! Neither my husband nor I wanted to go through it all again. We couldn't face the expense, the invasion, the threats to my health. But if something came along without intervention, well, that was definitely God's way. I now have two little girls and my baby son. I find it all hard to believe sometimes!

✼

A Final Word

Remember the good news: miscarriages don't always have to happen, if you know what tests should be done, what treatments are available, and what you can do yourself to help. Soon enough you will be holding that healthy, lovely baby you have been dreaming of for so long, a baby who will complete your family and bring much happiness.

RESOURCES

❦

Emotional Support Group Websites

American Fertility Association
http://www.theafa.org
This site deals with fertility and pregnancy loss.

Bereaved Moms Share
http://members.aol.com/BrvdMomShr/
Christian support group for mothers who have lost babies to miscarriage and stillbirth. To join, please send an e-mail to mailto:bereaved momsshare-subscribe@topica.com. You will need to send a letter of introduction about yourself and your losses.

Center for Loss in Multiple Births (CLIMB)
http://www.climb-support.org
An international website for couples who have experienced loss of a multiple birth.

The Compassionate Friends

http://www.compassionatefriends.org/

A national nonprofit, self-help support organization that offers friendship and understanding to families who are grieving the death of a child of any age from any cause.

Hannah's Prayer

http://www.hannah.org

Christian infertility and pregnancy loss group.

Hygeia

http://www.hygeia.org

This is an online journal for pregnancy and neonatal loss. It includes support information and links, individual stories, FAQs, and a downloadable booklet entitled "A Guide to Coping with Miscarriage."

IVF Connections

http://www.IVFconnections.com

Information and support for people going through IVF.

Multiple Miscarriages

http://www.surrogacy.com/online_support/mm/

You can sign up to become a member of this listserv. To subscribe, please send an e-mail to mailto:tasc@surrogacy.com and put "Send an application" in the subject line, or fill out the online application form on the website. This is for women who have suffered more than one pregnancy loss. The site also offers a chat area for live discussion of issues and monthly virtual seminars.

National Share Office

http://www.nationalshareoffice.com/

For pregnancy and infant loss support.

Pregnancy After Miscarriage (PAM)

http://www.pamsupport.org/pam.php

This list is now available to support couples either trying to conceive or carrying a baby after any kind of pregnancy loss. Anyone who has been in this situation and wants to offer advice or support is also welcome! This is not the place to post horror stories. It should be kept as a warm, fuzzy haven for getting questions answered and sharing concerns.

Resolve National Home Page

http://www.resolve.org/

The site includes listings of state chapters for pregnancy loss support.

Sidelines

http://www.sidelines.org

Offers support for patients who are on long-term bed rest.

Tefilat Chana

http://www.tzintz.com/atime

Jewish infertility and pregnancy loss group.

Medical Information Websites

International Council on Infertility Information Dissemination (INCIID)

http://www.inciid.org/

For medical information on immunological testing for miscarriage. Includes a chat room and bulletin board providing support for those experiencing infertility and miscarriage.

Reproductive Medicine Program

http://www.repro-med.net

Dr Alan Beer, a reproductive immunologist, posts articles on multiple losses and hosts forums for answering questions on infertility and recurrent miscarriage.

Early Path Medical Consultation Services
http://www.earlypath.com/
Pathology services working for safer pregnancies. Information on pregnancy loss as well as a service that may be able to help provide answers. Dr Carrie Salafia also helps out on the pregnancy loss board on INCIID.

Recurrent Pregnancy Loss and Implantation Failure Program
http://www.givf.com/immunev.cfm
Genetics and IVF Institute. Medical information.

Recurrent Pregnancy Loss Testing
Lists tests and procedures that are a mixture of the common elements of a recurrent pregnancy loss workup, including immunological screenings.
http://www.milenova.com
http://www.riala.com
http://www.haveababy.com

Books

Centering Corporation. *When Hello Means Goodbye*, 1985.
Available from the Centering Corporation, Box 4600, Omaha, NB 68104. Tel: 402-553-1200. E-mail: CenteringCorp@aol.com.

Cohn, Janet. *Molly's Rose Bush*. Albert Whitman, 1994.
Great storybook for children.

Faldet, R., and Fitton, K., eds. *Stories of Miscarriage: Healing with Words.* Fairview Press, 1997.
Moving writings from both mothers and fathers; also available in a Spanish edition.

Friedman, R., M.D., and Gradstein, B., M.P.H. *Surviving Pregnancy Loss: A Complete Sourcebook for Women and Their Families.* Citadel Press, 1996.
An in-depth look at the physical and emotional aspects, with a section on husbands and other family. Some personal accounts, with a good resource list and bibliography.

McCann, Mary Ann. *Days in Waiting.* de Reyter-Nelson, 1999.
Gives encouragement to patients on bed rest. See also http://www.sidelines.org.

Moffat P., Wilkins, I., and Kohn, I. *A Silent Sorrow: Pregnancy Loss: Guidance and Support for You and Your Family.* Delta, 2003.
Support for this often unrecognized loss. Includes information on how men and women grieve differently and the management of their subsequent pregnancies.

INDEX

᛭